PRAISE FOR
Uncertain Fruit

"Rarely have the urgent demands of a woman's biological clock been so vividly described as in *Uncertain
Fruit*, a moving account of a lesbian couple's years of
struggle to acquire a baby to parent. When artificial
insemination fails, they begin the adoption process for
a newborn boy. Richly evocative prose recreates their
joyful days of bonding with the baby—only to have his
teenage birth mother reclaim him. The numbing grief
this loss causes the two women is also poignantly conveyed. Part of the sadness for the reader is knowing
that so many potentially endangered babies need the
safe and loving home life that Rebecca and Sallyann
longed to provide."

—Lisa Alther, author of *Swan Song*

"Rebecca and Sallyann have written an amazing and
powerful book. 'The greater the love, the more enveloping the grief,' they write in the epilogue, and that
could not be more true as you read about their life
together. They deftly weave the story of their attempt
at adoption through the various strands of their individual lives: how they met, how they fell in love, and
forming a family that included Rebecca's two sons. It's

a beautiful and heartbreaking tale all at once, and we are all the richer for it."

—Mark Redmond, author of *Called: A Memoir*

"*Uncertain Fruit* is a candid, unflinching look at a couple's struggle to have a child of their own. Chronicling their extensive journey through physically and emotionally debilitating fertility treatments, explorations of adoption possibilities, and the heartbreak of relinquishing a baby they thought would be theirs, this book will resonate with all couples who've faced the harsh realities of infertility. Rarely have authors been so honest about every aspect of their lives and their relationship, their motivations and expectations, and their mixed feelings about the extent to which this overwhelming desire has controlled their lives. By taking turns telling their story, moving back and forth in time and place, they have produced a skillfully woven narrative that only the two of them could have birthed."

—Linda Peavy, poet and co-author of *Frontier House*

"*Uncertain Fruit* is an attempt to make meaning in the face of tragic loss by two women whose love for a child is only rivaled by their deep love for each other."

—Joanna Tebbs Young, MA, MFA, author of
*Lilian Baker Carlisle: Vermont Historian,
Burlington Treasure*

UNCERTAIN FRUIT

A Memoir of Infertility, Loss, and Love

UNCERTAIN FRUIT

A Memoir of Infertility, Loss, and Love

Rebecca Majoya
Sallyann Majoya

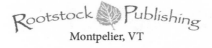
Rootstock Publishing
Montpelier, VT

First Printing: 2022

Copyright © 2022 Rebecca and Sallyann Majoya

All Rights Reserved.

Release Date: September 20, 2022

Paperback ISBN: 978-1-57869-097-8
Hardcover ISBN: 978-1-57869-098-5
eBook ISBN: 978-1-57869-099-2

Library of Congress Control Number: 2022903937

Published by Rootstock Publishing
an imprint of Multicultural Media, Inc.
27 Main Street, Suite 6
Montpelier, VT 05602 USA

www.rootstockpublishing.com

info@rootstockpublishing.com

Names and details in this book have been changed to protect the privacy of the people involved.

Book design by Eddie Vincent

Cover art by Candace Slack.

Author photo by Brian Farnum of B.Farnum Photography (bfarnumphotography.com)

"Autumn Sonnet" Copyright © by May Sarton, reprinted by the permission of Russell & Volkening as agents for May Sarton.

For permissions or to schedule an author interview, contact the authors at majoyawriting@gmail.com.

Printed in the USA

Dedicated to all of those we have lost along the way.
To those with a similar story, you are not alone.

If I can let you go as trees let go
Their leaves, so casually, one by one;
If I can come to know what they do know,
That fall is the release, the consummation,
Then fear of time and the uncertain fruit
Would not distemper the great lucid skies
This strangest autumn, mellow and acute.
If I can take the dark with open eyes
And call it seasonal, not harsh or strange
(For love itself may need a time of sleep),
And, treelike, stand unmoved before the change,
Lose what I lose to keep what I can keep,
The strong root still alive under the snow,
Love will endure—if I can let you go.

—May Sarton, "Autumn Sonnets"

PROLOGUE

If I can let you go as trees let go

FORFEITURE
Sallyann, 2015

I want to hate you, Delilah.
I want to hurt you, Delilah.
To dissect you like the frog coated in formaldehyde.

The formaldehyde of my middle school science class was pervasive and it hurt to breathe it in. All the room was covered in that chemical urine that coated the cold metal, and Ava was my partner for the frog. Its innards spread out on the metal tray before us.

She held the tools, the forceps. She made jokes. She always made jokes when she was uncomfortable. She had a gift for lightening the load that we bore together.

And there it was. There was a list and we had to figure out the parts. We had to lift each part onto a tray and cross it off the list just like that, as if the frog had never been.

It lay on its back with its legs splayed open, and we were in that cold room, starting the morning with the pungent compound and his cold amphibious frame, laughing.

And there was a heart.

I remember there was a heart once.

We pulled it out and it lay there next to him, as if it had never beaten.

And we laughed.

I didn't know how much I loved her then. I didn't love her like *that*.

We were awkward thirteen-year-olds, all gangly limbs, fresh periods, and greasy zits. We were pals who shared friends. We were little gigglers on the playground at recess.

We were mean. We laughed at the pimple-laden boy who took turns adoring us. We made fun of the way he walked. "Quack. Quack. Waddle. Waddle. Quack. Quack. Waddle. Waddle," we'd chant.

How could we be so mean? No regard for how much it hurt him.

But the playground was a vicious place for seventh- and eighth-graders. We were low in the pecking order. Other girls made fun of us and our differentness. Ava was the hand-me-down kid of five siblings. She wasn't dressed in designer jeans. She was a stumbler, a tripper, and, despite her dance training, it seemed she was still finding her way through space and her newly grown arms and legs didn't match up with the world around her.

She looked like a pixie or an imp. It was often hard to tell.

She reminded me of that fair-haired comedian, Ellen DeGeneres, whom I'd seen on late-night stand-up comedy shows. I thought the two of them should have been related. Even their jokes seemed to originate from the same writer: goofy, clean, and offbeat.

One-line zingers that pierced through the truth at the heart of the matter.

What was the truth?

Did I love her? Did I hate her? Did I want her, or want to be her?

But that was later on, when our relationship had brewed and steeped, then set in.

We were older and different somehow.

But with the lab in Mr. Colombo's science class, there was none of that complication.

I didn't feel all that then. Did I?

Or was it in there all along, the way lovers are in each other all along, as the mystical poet Rumi says?

Oh, of course I loved her. She was my best friend. Ava, Brooke, and I would traipse home after school, meandering through the park and having "wishy fights," blowing the white, puffy dandelion heads throughout the sky in some randomized competition that was not real. Or was real in the way only threesomes can be, competing for each other's attractions and desires.

But I didn't know desire *then*, not while the remains of the frog were spread out on the tin.

The desire came later.

It came when I returned from the absence of a move that had taken me 350 miles away. It came with the shared understanding of going to different schools from the rest of our friends. It came from the urgency and the excitement of reunion.

It came by surprise.

Hadn't we met in sixth grade? On the corner. Wasn't it Halloween? Brooke and I were trick-or-treating down the main street, and Ava was with a friend. Ava and Brooke recognized each other; their mothers knew each other from a Girl Scout camp they were in as kids.

Anyway, we'd bumped into each other before.

Maybe it was a chance meeting—a brief hello and introduction.

We never even gave a thought to it, or to the fact that we'd all be in the same school the next year.

And we didn't know then what we know now.

It's just a life mantra.

We didn't know then what we know now.

I remember it, though. It was my return to New Jersey from Vermont in our sophomore year, during the winter break. She'd blossomed. Ava was taller than me. It was as if all her limbs, which had languished, were now completely formed, and she had long legs, a dancer's legs, with those thicker muscular thighs perfect for jumping hurdles in track and field. Her features, her blond hair that she flipped with elegance and grace, all of it was beautiful. Not impish, but womanly, soft and strong—like her embrace.

When she hugged me, I felt her heart and her excitement. It zinged off me with the exuberance of a puppy. She had missed me and I was still her special person.

Our daily meetups in preparation for the upcoming New Year's parade were like little rendezvous in which we pledged our love and shared our thoughts. Oh, we were always good at sharing confidences, of ruminating deeply over the world, but we'd lost the silliness of the lab room and gained an intensity. We exchanged rings before I was to return to Vermont, and we wore those rings with a singularity and a purposeful passion.

The way you gave birth, Delilah.

I cried as he wriggled out of you in waves. I'd never seen this amazing, most wondrous process up close. My first introduction was in that eighth-grade science class with Mr. Colombo. It was on video, and it was something that was both fascinating and putrid, like the frog dissection. My peers left the class both awed and giggly, not sure what to do with all that blood and fluid and sexuality.

You pushed in silence and stillness with all your being, and we saw the crack in the sky from which his head emerged—a stump of dark hair that then sank back inside you, only to reemerge with the next heave-ho of your body and breath. He was more, then. More than a head. Soon he would be head and shoulders, knees and toes, rushing out on a wave and caught in the hands of waiting women. And there were not enough words, there never are, to describe all this wonder and all this love and beauty, and oh, all the desire and excitement and joy.

I held him against my skin, the little wonder, and he wriggled and moved and breathed and looked around. After all the fuss he had made as he entered this world, he was now the picture of peace. Silent and open, his eyes taking in the world, our arms enveloping him. At once I feared that I would never know how to handle him while also feeling as though handling him was the most natural thing in my life. Almost as natural as waking up or closing my eyes.

To hold a dream come true is beyond the scope of our language; it reverberates throughout the cosmos.

My little guy.

I never dreamed *I'd* have such a little guy. That we'd have *our* little munchkin, who was now naked against my naked chest, breathing against my heart, our hearts beating in harmony, in the wee small hours of the majestic morning in which you'd turned your head, kept your eyes closed, and released him to us.

Or so I thought.

Or so I'd hoped.

"Hope is the thing with feathers that perches in the soul." That's what Emily Dickinson says. But now hope was this living, breathing being we beheld. Our Sage boy, our little love muffin, my "smarmy" guy, the little pirate who'd stolen our hearts. A love unlike the others.

I loved you, Delilah. I think it was the moment we met you. I could not believe I was looking into the eyes of the person who would give me this gift of motherhood. I could not believe how hauntingly beautiful your eyes were, how adorable your features, and oh-my-god-how-fucking-young you were.

"Are you sure that you are old enough to carry that thing?" I wanted to say. "Aren't you twelve?" You looked sooo young and so innocent, so sweet and shy and scared. You had so few words to say and yet your eyes said it all. *Can I trust you?* they asked. *Will you take good care of this baby?*

They searched through my soul for all the answers.

For my part, I just wanted to shield you. You and the boy you came with. You were like little kids, and I felt this awesome responsibility to tread carefully, as well as to protect you.

Which is funny, really, because it was the same feeling I had when I held your beautiful creation, who had become my little boy. *My little boy.* I loved the way it sounded in my head and the way it echoed in my heart. *My little boy.*

I never imagined any of this. The room in the hospital, this precious baby whose birth I was part of. And Rebecca—how could I have ever imagined her, or the love I have for her?

I did imagine a future, back in the days of my sophomore year in high school. I imagined myself typing away at a novel. I imagined myself in a home with my successful husband. I imagined that I wrote while my first baby rocked quietly in a bassinet. I imagined that my first baby was a girl with brown eyes and brown hair and that she was the first of three babies that I would give birth to. I imagined her sweetness and her beauty, her big brown eyes, and her name. I imagined all sorts of things for my future. It kept me going through my long, dark, cold Vermont winter days, far away from people I loved and the familiar sights and walks and laughter.

At seventeen, what do you imagine for your future, Delilah? Is it really as little as you let on? You couldn't even answer—beyond where you were in life. At what point did you reveal an interest in traveling? It was as far into the future as you could go. Your world was so small.

We wanted to enlarge the picture for you. We wanted to give something back to you for all you were giving us. We wanted to alleviate our apprehensions and distill our guilt.

Oh, what was there to feel guilty over? We were not taking this away from you.

You were willingly giving it.

But how could you willingly give over what you don't even know you are giving?

You were not there with me at seventeen, Delilah, when I wanted to die because I realized I might actually be in love with her, with Ava, and if so that must have meant I was gay, and if I was gay that must have meant I'd never have those three beautiful babies I dreamt of, imagined holding and raising and loving.

What purpose did my life have if I could not be a mom?

It was all I wanted, besides being a writer. I wanted to be a mom.

I knew it was in every ounce of me and who I was. And I certainly did not want to be—oh, I could hardly utter the word, it was as sickening as the smell of formaldehyde: *gay*.

And I did not want to—I never imagined falling for her!

How did it happen?

Why did it happen?

Why me? Why now? What did I do wrong to deserve this punishment?

I must have done something wrong. I must be all wrong.

What is the purpose of my life now? Why am I here?

Maybe I *shouldn't* be here.

Did you have these thoughts, Delilah?

Maybe you had them when you found out that you were pregnant.

Maybe you had them after you were raped. (Or at least that's what you and Corey told us, and why disbelieve you?)

But what if you didn't have those thoughts?

What if you didn't reflect that much?

What if you thought you could have it over with, be done for good with the whole mess?

Or what if you were playing us all along? Stringing us along in hopes of having someone else who could care about the baby.

I want to hate you.

I want to strip your name and your being from my life.

I want you to disappear as if we'd never met, by coincidence or by the many teeny-tiny filaments that bring together lives in a strange and utterly impossible design. If you disappeared, if I'd never known you, maybe I wouldn't be feeling these horrible feelings, this confusion, and this pain. I wouldn't carry you in my thoughts and dreams. I wouldn't wonder how you were on a daily basis and want to reach out and connect, even as I want to damn you for putting me, putting *all of us*, through this.

PART ONE

If I can come to know what they do know

CHERYL'S CALL
Rebecca, 2014

The cell phone rings but I don't pick it up. I never do if I don't recognize the incoming call. I am enjoying the ride in our SUV with my feet on the dash. It is a mild fall day for October in Vermont, and I am just as happy to look at the turning leaves and relax. A minute later the ping sounds. Hmm, they left a message. *Stranger or friend?* I wonder.

"Sallyann, can you turn down the radio while I listen?" My hearing isn't great, and I recently acquired hearing aids, but interference can still be a problem.

I listen intently.

"It's Cheryl," I say to Sallyann. "She has a *situation* at school to talk to us about. Must be about another kid with autism or Asperger's." Our younger son, Seth, was diagnosed at age nine with Asperger syndrome, and Cheryl, a special educator, has often used us as resource parents to help de-escalate families who are overwhelmed with their child's behaviors or educational plan. It doesn't hurt that Sallyann and I have taken years of parenting classes and have been in individual and couples therapy. Working on our own shit does help us to help others sort theirs out.

I am always happy to assist Cheryl. She was a fabulous advocate for Seth when she was part of our school district and he needed services. She reminded us that some people in the education system *get it*—they understand us as parents, that we just want the best for our kids, unlike some educators who think we want our child coddled or given things that are unreasonable.

"I'll give her a call if you don't mind, sweetie."

"Sure, go ahead." Sallyann smiles.

I dial expecting to leave a message, but Cheryl immediately picks up the phone.

"Hello there, Rebecca. Is Sallyann there, too?" Cheryl sounds cheerful.

"Yes, sure. Do you want us on speakerphone?"

"Yes, please! I have some possibly exciting news for you."

Exciting? Hmm, not what I anticipated. Sallyann slows the car and pulls over into the parking area of a grocery store.

"So, there is a situation at the school with a seventeen-year-old girl. She is pregnant."

I freeze inside, goose bumps on my arms.

This is not the conversation I thought it would be. Not at all.

Cheryl knows we have been trying to adopt. She and her husband struggled with having children of their own, and had adopted a preschooler from foster care. At least a year ago, we met with her to talk about that situation, how it had worked out with her newest addition to the family. She could relate to us about the grief of infertility and was candid when discussing the process of adopting her little one. I felt Cheryl was a confidant, a friend on the level, not one who would ask for anything she didn't really need from us, so I wanted to help her out if we could. But that wasn't why she called.

"So, her mom wants her to keep the baby—the grandma, that is—but she told her special education teacher she thought she might just leave it at the hospital. She has said she would have aborted it if she had known she was pregnant in time, but she didn't," Cheryl explains.

"Wow, she must be under a lot of stress," I comment.

My many years of experience working for the women's shelter make me aware of how laden that statement is about her and her mom having different plans.

"So, I know you two are looking to adopt; I thought about you immediately."

"Is she interested in adoption?" Sallyann asks hesitantly.

"Yes, she said she is. I told her I know a couple, both women, who would be great parents, and she's interested in meeting you," Cheryl says.

"Does she have an agency she is working with, Lund or something?" I ask, referring to the state adoption agency we had registered with after deciding we were too nervous to go the foster care route. In foster care, we learned, it could take eighteen months or more for a baby to be released for adoption. Until the state deems the course impossible, the focus is on reunification with the family of origin. Sallyann and I could not imagine spending that long with a baby and then going through the process of turning them back over to the birth parents.

"No, and she doesn't want to. She is very private and just doesn't want a lot of people knowing her business, as she puts it," Cheryl says.

"Would we meet at the school? Alone with her, or with you or her special educator?" Sallyann is thinking to ask about details, while I am a bit dumbfounded.

"Yes, definitely," Cheryl responds. "If you're interested, I will see when we can meet. She is due the beginning of November, so there's only a few weeks before the baby is here. Oh, it's a boy. Is that okay?"

I look at Sallyann, she nods and then answers, "Yes, of course that's okay."

"Cheryl," I ask, "do you know if she has been doing drugs or alcohol while she's been pregnant?"

"She says she hasn't been, but I do think she drinks and most likely smokes, so I am not really sure. I guess we really won't know until the baby is here."

We look at each other; I can see the excitement in Sallyann's eyes. My own heart is beating a bit faster, with thrilled caution.

"Well, we can at least meet with her. What do you think, Sallyann?"

"Yes, tell her we'll meet and go from there."

We hang up, but my mind is abuzz. Is this real? We had been in the Seattle area visiting friends for a week and returned a few days ago. My brain had been fantasizing about moving west or south, not staying in the north. I was so damn sick of scraping ice off windows and shoveling snow. A warmer climate was calling me. We had been lightly talking about the baby search being not necessarily our calling anymore. It had been over eight years since we began fertility treatments. We were exhausted by it. All the ups and downs of the various methods we attempted in reaching for a baby to be left holding empty sleepers and an emptier bank account. Just a week ago it felt as if we were moving on to another place in our lives.

Now it is as if a baby is the only future possible. My body feels a pulsing energy at the thought of a tiny baby in our arms. It is as if the baby is here, as if we need to run to the nearest department store for diapers and onesies right this minute. The mind, it can toss you about like a ship on the sea. We were calm at the dock five minutes ago, with nothing pressing but what to have for dinner. I am torn between total glee and disbelief.

"So, you are okay with a boy?" I ask Sallyann again. We had listed our preferred gender as a girl on our paperwork for the adoption center. I knew she really wanted any healthy baby, but we'd both raised boys, and we were looking for the experience of another gender.

"Of course—we are great with boys." She smiles as she says it, and squeezes my hand.

"Yes, we are." I add, "Perhaps we are just meant to raise great boys into wonderful men." I squeeze her hand back.

DECIDING ON A WEDDING
Sallyann, 2005

We clinked our wineglasses against our friends'. The sound of Karen's booming voice carried across the table, seemingly across the room. "Happy V-Day!" she announced, and turned to her wife, June. "And happy anniversary!" She looked at her like a cat who'd swallowed a mouse. Since Karen joined the board of the women's shelter where Rebecca worked, we'd been clinking glasses of wine with these two quite a bit. Within the small population of our region, it was a relief to find another pair of lesbian professionals to hang out with. Karen, a corporate lawyer, and June, an insurance agent, liked to play as hard as they worked. They had invited us to join them on leisure trips to casinos in Connecticut, for boat rides on Lake Champlain, at their holiday party where two sips of the expensive wines they treated us to turned me tipsy. In exchange for their company, for regaling us with these outings, we'd dog sit their skittish sheltie whenever they took weekends away, or we'd provide our gardening skills for their landscaping.

Since we were celebrating their anniversary, Karen and June were recalling to us the details of their actual wedding ceremony in Massachusetts, where gay marriage had finally been made legal. It topped off their civil unions in two different states. They were on a mission to unite in every state they could, and it seemed that, like us, they'd found an anniversary for every occasion. I admired the giant rock on June's hand; fancy things were part of how Karen showed off her prizes. Karen nodded toward the diamond on my right hand. "So I see you have a ring, too, but you guys haven't gotten civil unioned yet, have you?" I looked sideways at Rebecca.

"It's been legal here in Vermont for several years now, and you've been together at least that long, right?" With Karen, I could always expect a cross-examination. I nodded.

"*So?*" She looked over at Rebecca, expecting her to answer the question that she originally posed to me. "So, when are you going to get married?"

I shuffled uncomfortably in my seat. Karen was as traditional as she was gay. She liked her life to follow a tidy, neat order and expected others to follow suit. I wondered if it compensated for the meandering life of the military brat that she'd lived.

Rebecca piped up. "I've left that concern up to her. I've already done the wedding thing. I've been married before. It's never been that important to me to do it all again."

I affirmed Rebecca's response. "Actually, it's never really been an issue for us. I mean, we've discussed doing it as a formality but I have not felt the need to declare my love in that way. We are already united. We're monogamous. We've created our own contract and we honor it. We did that before we moved in together."

I did not add that I'd seen plenty of poor representations of marriage, that I was not convinced that I needed special recognition to create a healthy marriage. My union with Rebecca belonged to us. We didn't need to flaunt it.

"Well." Karen shrugged. "Why the ring, then?"

Immediately, Rebecca took up the defense, smiling demurely at me. "Oh, I gave that to her for Christmas, early on in our relationship, because I wanted her to know that she was a gift of love in my life."

"You mean to tell me that you gave her an engagement ring and *didn't* have marriage expectations?" Karen was incredulous.

"It wasn't given with a date attached. Rebecca was showing symbolic commitment to me, but . . ."—again I shifted my weight—"she knew I was not looking to be married. We can still love each other without all the other conventional trappings."

I watched June nod knowingly. She, too, had been married before. She'd walked away from that heterosexual component of her life, told us that she felt freed from its constraints, only to uphold its appearances again with Karen.

"But what about your *kids*?" Karen was not going to let this drop.

Knowing her, I half expected a surprise wedding cake to be delivered from around her shoulder. I started wondering if she and Rebecca had been in collusion about setting up an engagement. But it was uncharacteristic of our relationship for Rebecca to discuss any decision related to us as a couple with someone else before she flew it by me, unless there was a surprise attached—and Rebecca was not good at containing secrets. She was so forthright that her every expression and emotion decorated her surface like a bumper sticker, in contrast to Karen's consistent poker face.

Karen continued, "Don't you want any legal protections for them? Or what about benefits?"

Rebecca eyed Karen curiously. "What about them? As domestic partners, we've been entitled to each other's health insurance in the state already. What would a civil union do that would be any more solid than what we've already created for the boys?"

"And Karen," I jumped in, "you know as well as we do that a civil union does not entitle us to half the benefits of a hetero married couple. The Feds don't recognize us. We can't file taxes together even though we pool all our resources. We can't expect to receive the other's social security benefits. If we were government employees, we wouldn't be able to receive the other's pension. That's all out of the question."

I turned the questioning on her: "Why did *you* marry?"

She smirked, reaching over to quickly grab June's hand. It was a brisk touch, one that would not stick long, as I could tell that Karen was uncomfortable with this public display of affection. As I watched the gesture in silence, I understood. Even in the progressive state of Vermont, I was still policing my external behavior with Rebecca. Being conscious of my every movement had been second nature to me since high school.

Where were we? Who were we with? Was it safe?

By not touching, were we complicit in the discomfort or even hatred of others? By touching, was our intent to genuinely connect? Would it be seen as trying to prove something?

It was June's opportunity to chime in again. "Well, for obvious reasons, I mean, right? For why anyone gets married. For love."

"And," Karen added excitedly, "because we actually *can* marry. People have been fighting for that right for eons, for the ability to be married and recognized and respected for their unions. Now we actually can."

I assessed her point.

I didn't need paper proof of my devotion to Rebecca and the boys. I knew that my legal rights to the boys were never unequivocal anyway, and a civil union would do nothing to change that. I couldn't adopt them. Their dad would not release his parental rights, and I would not ask that of him. But I wanted us to move forward. I would be thirty next year. Maybe I *should* reconsider this, especially if we decided to add to our family. As the banner of the women's rights movement stated, the personal was political. I could not ignore that. Yet I would not marry Rebecca to make a point to the state or Feds, to become a number in their census. As June said, I would do it for the obvious reason. To celebrate our love. To recognize it formally in front of friends and family. To share this occasion with the boys and with each other. To create our memory.

On the ride home that night, Rebecca and I continued where Karen left off, discussing the pros and cons of getting married. As much as we adored hearts and flowers, we were practical people. We weren't going to proclaim our love over a loudspeaker or stream it on a banner behind a dirigible.

As the night wore on, however, we warmed to the idea of a wedding occasion—even though it was still legally referred to as a civil union, which we reminded each other was separate from marriage. The event expanded around us, taking on a life of its own, until we agreed in bed: "Let's do it."

"But when?" Rebecca asked. I could see the dollar signs racking up in her eyes, the cost of a wedding overwhelming her more than the thought of marrying me.

"I like even numbers," I announced, "so I think we should wait until next year."

I jumped out of bed, heading in the direction of the calendar attached to the closet door. "How about June twenty-fourth?" I asked her.

She looked at me as if I'd just pulled a rabbit from a hat.

"Do you even know what day of the week that is?"

While she was asking, I was already flipping through the months. I looked up from the calendar and grinned.

"What?" Rebecca eyed me diligently.

"It's a Saturday."

"Well, I guess it's meant to be, then."
"Well, I guess it is."

MEETING DELILAH,
Sallyann, 2014

She doesn't want to meet us at the school with the special educators.

This makes me uneasy, giving me a sense that I'm rocking wildly over brackish waters.

But Rebecca reminds me that Cheryl told us she is a private girl and she is doing something against her mom's wishes. She reminds me of the countless women she'd counseled in her days at the women's shelter and how, sometimes, especially in an initial meeting, they just wanted close quarters, not too much interference. I remember my anxieties when I'd once met with a victim's advocate. The fewer people I had to tell my experience to the easier it seemed to me.

I didn't want to be any more exposed than I already felt. I don't want this young woman, considering us as potential parents of her soon-to-be baby, to feel any more uncomfortable than she already does. How bad could it be if we arranged to meet up at a public place in town? We are two adults. We'd worked in special education. While we have little idea what to expect when we meet her and do not know what issues made her eligible for special ed, we know we can handle it.

Besides, she might take one look at us and turn around.

Maybe she wouldn't come at all.

I feel overwhelmed. I have just returned to work after a trip to Seattle and I have so much to catch up on, so much planning to do, and now I'm taking time away again to meet up with this person who is younger than my student workers at the college, this girl who might turn her baby over to us. And then the phone call comes on Friday, and we arrange to meet this girl on Monday. The weekend becomes crowded with our anticipation, which overthrows all other thoughts.

We decide that our meeting place will be the corner coffee shop in town. Rebecca and I arrive early, positioning ourselves at a round table, large enough to accommodate four people and close to the entrance. We stare through the windows that surround the glass door, fixated on every person who walks toward us. We know she will be arriving with her boyfriend. She'd asked if he could come, too, and we thought that made sense, especially if he is agreeing to give up this baby, as well. Again, we want to make her as comfortable as possible.

Will they show up?

We watch the digital numbers change on our cell phones, listen to the rumbling of silverware and ceramic mugs as nearby tables are bused. And then we see the pair. It *has* to be them. She is short and sturdy, in a wide, candy-apple red winter coat that covers her extended paunch, and he is a gangly string bean in an overused jean jacket carrying a skateboard under his arm. They sit down sheepishly in front of us, appearing as vulnerable and childlike as I am feeling. She keeps her hands in her pockets, her coat wrapped close to her like a security blanket. Her hair is dyed with a pharmacy-box red, muted in comparison to her coat, and her roots are revealed in a streak of light brown.

I comment on the red hair and coat, and she says red is her favorite color.

Rebecca says that red is her favorite, too. And, like Rebecca, Delilah bites the side of her cheek, holding on to it for dear life. I stare at her as she does this, wondering if it hurts worse with the lip ring piercing.

We chat idly, Rebecca and me doing most of the talking, trying to make them feel we are trustworthy adults. Rebecca offers to buy them a beverage, and the boyfriend, who had introduced himself as Corey, eagerly joins her in picking out something warm to hold in his hands. Delilah, on the other hand, requests a glass of water. I smile, feeling encouraged that she is not choosing some sugared-up super latte, as so many of her peers would. Maybe she has been taking care of herself. Even if she doesn't want this baby, she still cares about it, just as I hoped she would.

Corey eases into conversation with us, while Delilah chooses her words carefully, cautiously, or quietly observes. I watch the two of them with each other; it is clear they understand each other in the way of young lovers, and Corey, in his own way, is trying to be respectful of her. He often turns to her and asks, "Isn't that right, baby?" or refers to her as *my girl*—"My girl doesn't want to keep her baby. I think that's a good plan." We find out that he is not the biological father—that the bio-dad is not in the picture.

Corey later reveals that Delilah was raped, that she is not interested in keeping this reminder of both the young man who'd hurt her at a party and of her shame. Because Delilah is the shy one of the pair, I feel compelled to include her as much as possible, to ask her as much as she is willing to share. I also keep assessing her body language. Is this what she really wants? Does she seem certain? Does she like us? Would she choose us? How much does she care? How real is this to her?

Her eyes are a phlegmatic blue, resigned to hold back even as they want to be more curious. I find myself wondering if his eyes, the baby's, will resemble hers.

We spend over an hour with them before they leave to catch the bus—we learn that neither of them has a car or a license to drive. We find out that Corey dated Delilah in the past, that he is older than her, that he is on probation for minor possession of marijuana. We find out more about why Delilah wants to put her baby up for adoption and how little she wants to be a part of its life. We also learn that they have no problem turning this child over to gay parents. In fact, Corey adds, he has an aunt who is married to another woman.

I am enchanted by this young couple. We both are. They are brave. They want to do right by this baby. They want to give it a life that they admit they could not.

Yet we are still surprised when they agree to meet us there again the next day, agree to let us look into legal counsel for us both, shocked that they are choosing us. We agree to see them again tomorrow, when we'll review what we learn from the lawyer and continue to develop our relationship with them.

On the car ride home, I clutch Rebecca's hand. Could this be for real? It is like a fairy tale with a real live happy ending. But it is all moving so quickly—from a series of roller coaster rides into free fall.

DR. FITZPATRICK'S OFFICE
Sallyann, 2005

Here I was: Feet in stirrups. Flat on my back with an uncomfortably scratchy paper towel rolled flat beneath me. My legs were spread and, from this view, all I could see was his balding head and latex-gloved hands as he asked me to please scoot my butt further down toward him and the edge of the table. I commented on the adjustable stool he'd rolled over the tiles and settled before my pelvis. He acknowledged that it was new and much needed; as he got older he'd become aware of the importance of caring for his back.

He was a gentle doctor, tenderly placing his hand over my lower abdomen and announcing what I should feel. He was palpating around my uterus and ovaries from above before plugging into me with his digits to check everything from the inside. He asked how "Becky," my partner, was. He always called her by this familiar nickname, the same name her family of origin called her, the name she refused to go by as an adult. I never felt he was asking about my beloved, but about somebody I should know well enough to discuss while being touched in my intimate zones. He moved on to preparing the duck lips—the clamps that will spread my cervix and open me for a swab. So far, so good, as far as we were both concerned. I appreciated that he asked how she was doing, recognizing her importance in my life.

I thought about him as he had stood at the end of her hospital bed a little over a year before and told us the news about her fibroid, the giant mass that took over her abdomen and caused her to bleed incessantly, to go through a box of supersize tampons in a day. He advised emergency surgery once she was sufficiently pumped up with enough units of blood to burst the guts of a village of mosquitoes. We had no idea she had been this close to dire circumstances. We both blew it off as symptoms of early menopause and getting older. After all, she was going to be forty, and menopause was like adult adolescence. It caused the body to do all kinds of crazy things.

I sat on the hospital bed beside her with her hand in mine, aware of the warmth and the pulse I cherished so much. It was quick, the turnaround of events. She was anemic all those months we denied the level of her pain, the seriousness of it all. And she could have just dropped, she could've just . . .

I could not hold the thought for long. It was far more terrifying than the monsters in my childhood closet. This was real, it happened, and it moved fast, deciding our fates for us.

I remembered my college English professor, Dr. Dugan, standing at the front of the classroom in Wilson Hall, one of my favorite rooms in the exquisitely designed building, which was styled after a Louis XIV treasure. She was pacing as she spoke to us, her scarlet hair flying around her head. Like most of my best English teachers, her background was in drama, and we could never get through a class without her treating us like a participating audience. She walked into the classroom with stage presence, she huffed loudly, she touched her forehead emphatically, and she smiled broadly. She was telling us that our theme for the semester was the individual versus the community, and she planned to structure the class and our readings around the theme. Moreover, we were going to address another literary theme—fate versus free will. I sat up straighter in my chair, aware of the stillness in the class, the breathing of the students next to me. "Is it all fated to be?" she asked before pacing to another part of the room and looking directly into my eyes. "Or the results of the choices you make?"

Dr. Fitzpatrick was staring at me quizzically as if wondering where I'd gone or why I hadn't immediately responded to him. "Are you doing okay?" he asked, as he began inserting the speculum. "You seem pretty tense. Just breathe. That will make it easier."

I'm pretty sure I'd heard that a million times in my life. But didn't he know how difficult it was to breathe when searing pain was shooting up your body? I could sense his tension. I was not opening up easily. I stared at the ceiling. There was nothing there but blue paint. I could have used one of those rooms with a Caribbean

Sea poster or a fuzzy kitty looking down at me. Instead, I had blue paint under glaring fluorescent lights, and now he was doing his best to assuage my tension by asking me if it usually hurt like this, if I had trouble with sex because of it.

Really? Maybe he thought he was using his doctor skills to get me to talk and deliver some release of my pelvic muscles, as if I could breathe between words, then, voila! Before we knew it, he'd done the deed and pulled out. He didn't have a clue what sex was for "Becky" and me, and he wasn't comfortable asking.

When he had prepped for the removal of Rebecca's uterus, he did have the kindness and forethought to inquire whether she would want to keep her ovaries intact. And then he added, "I'm not exactly sure if this is important to you and your partner, since I'm not sure what you do for sex, but I can also keep your cervix intact, if you would like, if this matters to you sexually, in particular." He was doing his best to be politically correct, and we chuckled after he exited. What exactly *do* you lesbians do?

Now I could feel his ignorance once more as he endeavored to help me with my issue by telling me all about the importance of breathing practices that could help me loosen up those noncompliant muscles, as if I hadn't spent most of my life learning how to breathe.

It was time to sit up again and speak to each other on corresponding planes of space.

"Everything otherwise looked all right except for your tension. Any idea what may cause it?"

Besides the obvious? I thought.

"Well, you mentioned before the exam about my polycystic ovary syndrome and me being just past thirty. You said that, as of now, I couldn't have a baby without intervention."

"I can't prophesy," he said, "but it's simply that you're not ovulating. Without the release of the egg each month, the reality is that you won't be able to get pregnant with your condition unless you consider a course of treatment. I can recommend a specialist in Burlington. He can tell you more about the process and put you on an infertility treatment plan. As of now, your hormones are all messed up, out of balance. So you need to deal with that, of course."

I nodded and pulled my johnnie around me. He patted my shoulder reassuringly. I wondered if he could feel me wince.

"Just let me know what you decide," he said, with my file of medical information already under his arm, "and we can go from there."

HIRING THE LAWYER
Sallyann, 2014

Our friend Cathy recommends a lawyer in town, Irene Haines, whom she'd called upon years before in the adoption of Cathy's grandchild.

As we sit in Irene's office explaining our situation to her, requesting her skills, I can see her mentally checking off what she will need to take care of.

"On my end, there's not going to be too much, mostly paperwork, but you will need to hire the lawyer for the birth mother. From the sounds of it, you may require her intervention a bit more."

I like Irene. Her eyes are kind and betray her sophisticated, hardened legal facade.

"I will warn you that her fee is a bit more than mine. If she can do it, you will have a larger retainer to reckon with."

Anything. We'll pay anything.

Time was of the essence.

We met Delilah and her boyfriend, Corey, only yesterday. We know she is due in two weeks and that she wants to move forward with us. If we are going to do this, we need her lawyer on board to meet with her and get a real sense of what we are up against. Anyway, the fees for both lawyers have to be less than the more than twenty-five thousand dollars the adoption agency asked us to come up with.

"Okay," Irene says, shaking our hands after the retainer and her services have been agreed upon. "This is exciting news. I'm really looking forward to working on this adoption with you."

A couple of days later, once Irene and Jenifer—Delilah's lawyer—conferred over Delilah's situation, Irene advises, "This could go well. It's still hard to say, but"—she hesitates—"you will need to protect your heart, in any case."

Protect your heart? What does that mean? Surely I could've used the "Protect your heart" advice at other times in my life. It seems to make about as much sense as "Make your peace" with the person who'd caused you pain.

I'm pretty sure it's already too late for that, Irene, I think.

It's too late, baby. It's just too late.

I search my mind for examples of what it means to protect your heart. *Would the Dalai Lama advise this?* I think. Didn't Mother Teresa tell us to keep an open heart so it could bear the suffering of the world? All the spiritual words of others are wringing out, hanging to dry around me. Do they ever tell you to protect your heart? The only way I succeeded in doing that was with fear. According to *The Gift of Fear*, by Gavin de Becker, fear is an ally, there to warn us and take care of us. I am at odds with the notion that you could have an open heart while behaving from a place of fear, but I suppose that could be my daily approach to life. I thought about the heart's ability to take the bitter with the sweet. If anything, it seems that it's less about needing to protect our hearts from what might happen and more about protecting them from ourselves and our own expectations.

SPERM FOR SALLYANN
Rebecca, 2008

I wanted to have a baby with her.

Was that so wrong?

Because I am a woman, I could do nothing to help her.

I read about it in the paper every day. There were so many people who didn't deserve a baby that had one. People who neglected them, or abused them. There were people who popped them out like rabbits.

I just wanted to have a baby with Sallyann, and I couldn't.

I could not give her anything from me that would create a baby in her.

I could not, no matter how often or lovingly I made love to Sallyann, impregnate her.

I gave birth to two boys with my ex-husband, but now I was completely and desolately infertile. The emergency hysterectomy I'd had would not allow me to offer a womb to carry a child for us.

We sat up long nights in bed looking through hundreds

of sperm donor profiles. On that large, soft, king-size bed, we lay surrounded by six or more pillows piled up to comfortably lean against the headboard that supported us. Three cats, one on each side of the bed and one at our feet. The first choice was which donor bank to work with. Each had its own questions and features. Some would give only a minuscule amount of information if you didn't pay extra money per profile. There were long pages of questions with answers from prospective donors on health, education, and hobbies. How would we know if they were telling the truth? From the backgrounds given, most were college age and most likely doing this for the money, I thought, regardless of the flowery things they wrote.

So many decisions to make in the process, it was overwhelming and comical. What nationalities are okay? Height, weight, education level, hair color, eye color? What were their occupations and health risks? Are the donor's parents still living?

Then the more serious concerns. Do you want a donor who agrees to be known after the child is eighteen or one who wishes to be forever anonymous? We both believed in honesty, but it was also awkward to think of our child going off to meet a stranger—a stranger who shared their genetic code.

We laughed nervously as we flipped through online pages and paper pages sent our way from sperm banks coaxing us that these were the right fathers for making our dreams come true. Reading the answers to questions like *What would you want your child to know about your decision to donate your semen?* we often asked ourselves if maybe they were lying, if it was all just a big hoax. We looked through their lists of achievements at Ivy League schools, their great athletic prowess, the empty boxes where they could mark which defects run in their family.

Was it true? How could we know? But then, we both have blanks in our genealogy, too . . . so do we know what we would get if it was our own genetic code? Not really.

We looked at pictures of the donors as babies and as adults, depending on the website. Some offered videos of a donor answering questions so we could hear his voice.

It was surreal, this choice.

I stood next to Sallyann while they poked and prodded her with various instruments, while she took medicine by mouth and by injection to get the eggs to ripen. Then I held her hand while they stuck in the long tube to inseminate her with a stranger's sperm.

Not mine; nothing from me. I could not give my blood to her, or anything to help out.

MEETING DEBBIE
Sallyann, 2014

"My mom would like to meet you," Delilah states politely. We are on day two of our meetings, and Delilah has requested that her mom join us the next time we meet. In the next breath, she arches her brow at Corey in response to his grunting noise. "She's *not* crazy."

"I can't stand her mom," Corey says to me as we order his coffee at the front counter. Of course I want the opportunity to meet this baby's biological grandma. Yet Corey's words at the counter make me feel wary. "We argue all the time. Her mom is so selfish and self-centered. It's all about her. She will do anything she wants because she only cares about herself." He winces as if he's stubbed his toe. "She didn't even believe it when Delilah told her she was raped. Can you believe that? She thought she was making it up. She laughed it off. Why would she do something like that? What kind of mom treats her daughter like that?"

Listening to him, I ponder what side of the story I am hearing. He's made it clear since we met the day before that he has no positive feelings for the birth father, someone he'd once been friends with. He told us that the birth father was into selling drugs, and that this young man's mother sold heroin from their house, none of which surprised me. I was well aware of the opioid abuse problem that had been wreaking havoc in our community. But, without having met Delilah's mom, I try to withhold judgment. I consider that maybe Corey, a young man diagnosed with ADHD, who is also on probation, was simply not approved of by her mother, that whatever he has to say about her is the reaction to her mother's disdain for him. Before we leave, we agree to meet Delilah's mom. I ask Delilah what her mother's name is and mentally record it.

That night, my curiosity getting the best of me, I look for her mom on Facebook. I don't see much on her page, but her profile picture is exceedingly familiar to me.

"Rebecca." I nudge her as I indicate the photo. "Do you know her? It doesn't look like we have any mutual friends. But I remember her. I think she worked at Grand Union—or maybe it was Price Chopper—back in the day." There is something about her demeanor, even in that photo, that is unforgettable to me.

"Oh my gosh," I say, noting the birthdate on her page. "She's younger than me, too. She must have been a young mom herself when she had Delilah."

"That's very likely, too," Rebecca responds.

She is intrigued but is also busily folding the new baby clothes we picked up from the outlet store tonight. We are already so excited, we are bursting at the seams. We can barely wait to put those itsy-bitsy onesies on our soon-to-be baby. Do we really have to wait a couple more weeks? My gut keeps telling me it will be sooner. Much sooner.

Once again, we sit at the table near the front entrance of the coffee shop. This time, I watch as a wiry-haired woman with icy-cool eyes bounds into the space ahead of Delilah and Corey. She puts her hand out and shakes ours with distant formality, then plops down at our table next to Delilah, who is shut up like a clam in its shell.

I try to be open, try not to meet her mom with the suspiciousness she seems to emanate.

I consider her features, how she is younger than me but looks considerably older, as if life has eroded her around the edges. It is a mild day in late October, and she wears a tank top that barely covers her ample cleavage. Along her arm is a bleeding snake tattoo, and on her neck she proudly displays to us her recent tattoo of a cleaver, also dripping blood. At another time, I might have been intrigued by her, might have discussed her passion for horror movies with her. After all, I grew up with a mom who devoured horror novels and sci-fi movies. My mom was enamored with vampires, Frankenstein's monster, bogeymen. Debbie brags about her collection of zombies and Chucky dolls, about her six-year-old daughter's fascination with all things black, morose, and bloody, about how they are so excited to celebrate the upcoming Halloween.

Rebecca and I love Halloween, too. We consider it one of our most celebrated holidays, but we are uncomfortable with anything that is too visceral, too much like real life. We prefer goofy ghosts, cackling witches, plump pumpkins, mysterious black cats.

Debbie does not leave much to mystery. She doesn't leave much space for anyone else, for that matter. She speaks nonstop, but not in a nervous way, more to dominate the conversation.

I ask if she'd ever worked at Price Chopper, and she confirms that she'd worked her way to assistant manager a while ago, but left the job after some problems with a boss and the death of a family member. She does not seem surprised that I recognize her, as if she is used to being a local Price Chopper celebrity. She announces that she is furthering her education, taking advantage of the Reach Up program to attain her bachelor's degree through the state college.

"Oh, really? What in?" I ask, and before I even finish the question, she launches into the details of her program in social work, how she is nearly done with her clinical requirements, would have been finished "if not for interruptions like the death of my mother and having to deal with a pregnant seventeen-year-old."

"But," she adds, "when I'm done with this degree, I don't really care if I do social work. I don't really want to work. Maybe I could just bag groceries." She snickers.

I can tell she is savvy enough not to make that declaration at a job interview, that she would do whatever she needed to survive; but I can't tell if she is trying to be off-putting, to play into some kind of welfare stereotype, or to push our buttons to see what we find humorous.

"I can't believe that you two have never met before," I say, gesturing to Rebecca and Debbie. "You know,

Rebecca's been in social work for over twenty years."

Rebecca asks Debbie where she is interning, and Debbie responds "with United Way," an organization Rebecca has frequent contact with. For such a small area, it is remarkable that their paths have not crossed.

As if not wanting to share what she might have in common with Rebecca—with either of us—Delilah's mom moves abruptly on to other topics. She tells us that she lives right in town but hates it, that she'd grown up in the country and wanted to return there, to be "away from people." She reminds us that she has to be in town, close to the elementary school where her precious Eloisa goes. She makes no mention of the seventeen-year-old sitting next to her as she launches again into a story about the six-year-old who takes up so much of her energy.

When we finally return to the reason we are there, Rebecca asks how she feels about Delilah's wishes to give up the baby. "Well, you know how teenagers can be, and Delilah has a mind of her own. She thinks she can do whatever she wants."

When we ask further, she shrugs. "She can do what she wants. She knows that."

Delilah told us the day before that she will not be reachable by cell phone much longer, that her dad stopped paying for it. When we ask if Debbie is concerned that Delilah will be without a phone, that she might be couch surfing in another part of town—as she and Corey told us they've been doing—when she goes into labor, Debbie shrugs again.

"I barely see her as it is. Most likely, I'll hear she is in labor from Mimi." She laughs derisively and shifts her eyes toward Delilah, as if giving her some inside jab. She informs us that Mimi is her younger sister, just seven years older than Delilah. Apparently, Mimi and Delilah are close.

Debbie takes another jab at her teenager. "Mimi's pregnant, too. She's due in March. So, at least I will get to hold *her* baby."

"You know," we add, "we can send pictures if you'll give us your email address. And it's not like we are very far away. I'm sure you will see him around." The thought of having more contact with this woman sends my stomach into somersaults. The whole time we are together she barely lets Corey or Delilah get a word in edgewise. She fills the air with words just to take up space. I want badly to believe that she is supportive of her daughter's choices to "do whatever she wants," but it is difficult to believe, especially when her volume is turned up so much higher.

We volunteer to take Delilah to the store to purchase a TracFone and calling card, so she at least has a way to communicate during this time that labor is imminent. We all get up and march over to the local pharmacy, to the cell phone department, where Debbie hovers over Delilah, interjecting as if Delilah has no ability to make the decision. I back up and bite my lip. I can see that Delilah is used to letting her mother decide for her, letting Debbie treat her as if whatever is in her head is not as smart or as capable as what is in Debbie's. How can I pay attention to anything but the jumping jacks Debbie's behavior sets off in my belly?

INSEMINATIONS
Sallyann, 2008

I've never been a fan of hospitals but even less so when I'm lying on my back, feet hoisted up in stirrups, legs spread wide open. I was alone this time. Rebecca couldn't be here but, really, it was just another checkup and check-in. Another probing and prodding to assess the state of my eggs. Have they been released yet from their chambers?

I thought about my egg compartments, my little ovaries. I wondered if they had felt abandoned by me, if my younger self felt abandoned by me.

After all these years, you're finally trying, and trying, and trying to produce one baby. Oh, I hoped this baby's struggles would be easier than my own, easier, moreover, than the generations' before me.

There's something so pricelessly scientific, seeing the gel on the ultrasound probe. But that science was crippled by the emotions I felt when the probe slid its way into me and I was aware of the cold and heat, of the fear and discomfort of my body. There were two screens in the room on which to view my ovaries, not that I could make much out of the picture unfolding. I felt the pressure of the probe against my pelvis. The physician apologized for the pressure as he tried to take pictures. He was not my usual doctor, and his bedside manner was hardly comforting. He talked about me, over me, to the technician who was with him. They discussed something in relation to my eggs as if I was not even there, but I was sure I was in my body this time. I could feel everything that was within me.

They took measurements of each follicle, assessing the ripeness: fifteen centimeters, not quite ripe enough. They counted at least three that, by their standards, looked quite good. I will need to drive the 140-mile trek, another four hours two days from now, before we can go through with the next insemination, Mr. 6677. Wasn't it strange to think about this unknown intentional bio-father as if talking about a version of a robot, about C-3PO?

I was okay now with the fact that my baby daddy was not holding roses for me, or a drink. He wasn't spouting off his latest idea, or ruminating over the world with his coffee and newspaper. That is, while he could have been doing all these things and more somewhere on this Earth, he was not doing them with or for me.

There was a time I'd thought differently. I had believed in the ideal conception, all hearts and flowers, all emboldened by love. I had believed in the love of a man and a woman uniting to create the majesty and miracle of an Earthling.

I had believed that was the only option. And I wanted so badly to experience that.

But it was much more of a playful idea, like pretending as a little girl to marry my Muppet Scooter doll. It was a grand wedding for Scooter—I called him John—and me.

I donned my best dress and my veil, and carried him down the green indoor-outdoor carpeting of my bedroom, so proud of our devotion to each other. I even requested a photographer to commemorate this holy day. I was in love with Scooter John, and he was enthralled with me, and together we would live just like the fairy tales, happily ever after. We hadn't talked children then, Scoot and I, but it was a given. After all, everyone knew the playground chant, and I had already checked off love and marriage. Obviously, next would come the baby carriage.

I picked myself up off the table. The doctor was done with me. I could wipe the remnants of cold gel from around my inner thighs and dress my lower half.

I was beginning to wonder if this would ever take. Thank goodness for age. It was allowing me to lose track of the years I was spending in this process.

It was age that was also keeping track of my follicles, parceling them out like an Easter egg hunt.

I'd spent most of my life feeling as if there were a spotlight over my head and a ticking clock sounding beside it.

On the way out of the hospital, as I was handing over

my parking ticket, I was surprised to realize I'd been there for such a short time that I didn't need to pay for this visit. I thought about the humor of my situation. Most of my job, even my day, was spent planning the next event, the next meeting, the next month, the next year. I could plan for all my job required of me, but I could not plan for a baby. They happened of their own accord. All spotlight. No watch.

ROXIE AT THE PUB
Rebecca, 2014

The live Irish music fills the pub as we chat with our good friend Roxie about our adoption plans. I order another Corona with double lime and tell her about the crib we've just set up, describing the process by flailing my hands in demonstration of the useless instructions.

"Wow, you guys are really serious!" she remarks in the dim light of the dark wood-paneled room.

"Yes, if you can survive putting a crib together, then you're going to be able to parent together, right?" I smirk.

"I'll drink to that." She lifts her Guinness.

We laugh even though we have been parenting together for twelve years, and trying to add to our family has been anything but funny. We laugh so often when we want to cry.

"How are the boys about it?" she asks, as we pound the table in rhythm to "Whiskey in the Jar" on the fiddles and drums.

"Well, Seth is thrilled." Sallyann immediately fills her in. "Sawyer . . . he is in his own geekdom. As usual, he is fine as long as it doesn't rock his world."

"Right. The 'does it change anything for me?' deal.

That's his gig."

"Typical college-age reaction," Sallyann adds, and excuses herself to visit the ladies' room.

As soon as she is out of earshot, Roxie begins: "So, tell me how you *really* feel. You can't want another baby. You're fifty years old!"

I don't know what to say. I look toward the bathroom where Sallyann had disappeared, as if she could help me somehow explain from afar.

"Yes, I do really want this. Why would I pretend about something like this? I mean, it is a lifetime commitment, another child. How could I fake that? Why would I? That would totally suck for our relationship."

"Yeah, but have you thought it through? Diapers all over again, the late nights, and getting up in the night. You are free of all that. You could do anything."

"Yes, and I want *most of all* to be happy with Sallyann. She has been trying for so long. Why wouldn't adoption be the next step?"

"When she started trying it was almost eight years ago, though. You were forty-two then, for crying out loud."

"Now I'm fifty. I have good genes. My people live— we live a long time. I'm talking mid-nineties."

"What about the cost? You're still paying for the boys' college?"

"Yep, and this will cost about the same as what we owe for the two of them together. So I guess this little one better find scholarships, just like the other two!" I laugh and take another chug of my Corona. Seeing our low glasses, a waitress comes by and pauses.

"Yes," Roxie confirms. "Give us another round."

At least that is one good thing with adoption—not carrying a child, I can drink.

And I need it right now.

I have never been so grateful to have my wife return from the bathroom.

I put my arm around her as she takes her seat at the rustic wood table coated with many layers of polyurethane. "I can't imagine not taking the chance to raise a child with this woman. This time, being able to do what we see as best without worrying about *dad's* reaction to everything. The boys have been the most frustrating, delightful, and crazy part of my life. And I'm game for more!"

"I'll drink to *that*." And we all raise our glasses and clink.

I try not to think of my age. I know our family has great genes. I also know anything can happen at any time, so it isn't about age, is it? It is more about doing what you love and living life, isn't it? I hope so. I think I am up for this. I believe I am. That's all we have, isn't it? Lots of hope.

I remember seeing Sallyann for the first time. I met her in a little holistic health store. It was called Peace of Mind. For real, you couldn't make that up.

I knew Peace of Mind carried gifts and cards because I'd been there a few times before, but it had been a while. I never believed in love at first sight, until that moment. I saw her and I knew it *was* a real thing, that you can see someone and feel you have known them your entire life, maybe more than a lifetime. As soon as I walked in, there she was, standing behind the long counter in front of a collection of boxes and ribbons for gift wrapping.

"I need a gift," I stammered. "A gift for someone getting married that you think is making a very bad decision." I joked, without including that the gift was for my ex-girlfriend who had cheated on me with an unauthorized immigrant. She was marrying him to help him get a US green card so he could stay in the country since she was pregnant with his child—her fourth—all within six weeks of cheating on me.

"I need something simple," I continued, more to allay the nervousness that had come over me than to convey the gift choice.

"Do you think you have anything inexpensive but thoughtful?" I added. It sounded cheesy the moment it was out of my mouth. For the next half hour, we walked around the store. I talked, she laughed, I laughed, and at one point, she blushed. I think I may have, too. We managed to find a little angel pin that fit the bill. She wrapped it, choosing the paper and ribbons so perfectly, I thought. So appropriately and sweetly making it look more majestic than the contents deserved.

I wanted to hug her when I left. I wanted to stay, but I was on my way to my second job at a restaurant up the hill. I explained my black-and-white apparel so she would understand this wasn't my desired attire, just what was demanded by my next hours of service. Why did I need to have her care about my clothing choices?

It was later that night when I knew I would be making many more trips to Peace of Mind.

I was staying with a fellow waitress friend, Paula, who lived in town, so I would have quick access the next morning to the restaurant. Closing at 11 p.m. and then opening for breakfast at 5:30 was how I got the most hours in and still met the demands of a single mom once my boys got home from time with their dad. Paula was whining about the bad dating scene post-divorce. Then she realized how horrid it must have been for me.

"How do you even know if someone is gay?" she asked at midnight, as we chattered off our waitressing buzz.

"I don't, I guess, any more than you know if they are straight!" We both laughed and sipped our wine. "But today I met the most beautiful woman, and I don't know if she is a lesbian or if she is single, for that matter."

This ignited Paula's imagination, and she had to know where I'd met her and when.

"Peace of Mind?" she exclaimed. "I go there for massages all the time. What was her name?"

"Sallyann. She was—"

"Not only do I know her, I just found out last week from my massage therapist that she *is* gay and she *is* single."

I was silent. Was this possible? Really?

Needless to say, I found lots of reasons over the next month to buy cards and work up my nerve to finally ask her out.

As I sit and drink another Corona, I can't believe it has been almost fourteen years since then.

"I guess I'm driving." Sallyann smiles knowingly at me. I take out my keys and hand them over, a pleasant buzz going.

"Yes, absolutely!" I stand up and declare. "Yes, baby mama, I guess you are the one in the driver's seat."

Roxie's look makes it clear she still thinks I am crazy.

The really crazy thing is, I don't even mind.

QUADRUPLETS
Sallyann, 2012

Sometimes I'd get so angry with myself. Why couldn't I be done with this whole baby thing already? Why did I have to insist on putting us through this? So many stupid years that felt wasted, traveling from doctor to doctor, from allopathic medicine to alternative healing. All those mornings I took my basal temperature, trying to glean any clue as to when I might ovulate, all the tests, all the worrying. Poor Rebecca had lived for years with the quietly insane, agitated woman whose nerves seem to be poking into both of us like broken underwires in a bra.

Even before the hormone treatments I was a bundle of edginess. I could not drive into the downtown without sniffing the diapers, witnessing the teenage girls pushing strollers aimlessly, not babysitting, but mothering instead. I wanted to stop them in their tracks. They were so preoccupied they did not even see the lights in front of them, flashing green, while each tapped away at her cell phone, more immersed in it than the infant ahead of her. They mocked me with their reckless fertility that was not within me, even though I had once believed it was.

In my younger years, I used to worry I'd get pregnant at the drop of a hat. It haunted me like an invasive weed that popped up in the most inopportune places. I used to think I was an effulgent garden, uterus just waiting for that magical science of ovum and sperm. Because I was fearful of potential pregnancies that could ruin my future, there was no way I was going near men. It wasn't as though I was ever on the prowl for a relationship, anyway.

Still, I felt nothing but shock that my basal temperature barely changed, and I worried over it being remarkably low. Why couldn't I ovulate?

Then, when I began fertility treatments and produced several healthy-seeming, ripened ova, I remember the feeling of being larger-than-life, carrying the ability to create it.

Rebecca and I would grow excited with anticipation after every round of inseminations. "I just know it's going to take this time," she'd say, committed to her faith that I had the baby-making powers within me and they were at work, basting my fallopian tubes and uterus, preparing me for the stuffing.

Then came the disappointment when it didn't take, when I'd perform yet another pregnancy test, staring excitedly at the little plastic wand, waiting for the little cross or Yes mark to pop up, and again I'd see another sign of my epic failure to breed. This was followed by Rebecca's crestfallen expression that mirrored my own emotions. *Back to the drawing board*, I'd think. I'm racing against the clock. I'm betting on the horse that may never win, aging daily, moving closer to death, and without a trace of life within me.

I appreciated Rebecca's enthusiasm each time it seemed that much more possible—just this time, just this once. But when she'd say she'd felt so sure it would work, so positive I would be pregnant, I'd feel my sense of failure again. It was all on me and I couldn't do it, the worst kind of ineptness. I visualized myself sitting on the edge of the bed while she comforted me in my inability to get it up.

"Maybe next time," she'd say.

But I knew that was the thing about fertility treatments. They were like our days on Earth: finite. You only had so much time and then you ran out. This only increased my anxiety. I read about how important it was to relax through the process, and I'd laugh sardonically. What a joke! As if most babies were created when the parents were not under stress, worried about how to pay the bills, keep a roof over their heads. The truth was that I could only embrace the uncertainty, or the certainty that it would never take. Either way, it was always a gamble, and the cards were less in my favor each time I played them.

We were in this together, too, which made me feel all the more selfish when I dragged us through the highs and lows, each time the fertility drugs gave me the feelings of a woman in early pregnancy, the warm glow of creation within me. And then—there it was again, the stopwatch.

I felt guilty even though she had agreed to go along with me, even though I watched as more layers of gray filled her hair, the gravitational forces of the years pulling her down. She remained exquisitely animated, but life was doing what it does, aging us both before our eyes, which was further corroborated by watching the boys grow beside us.

I thought of our friend Eva when Rebecca first announced to her that I was hoping to have a baby. Eva had one daughter, whom she cherished and doted over. She'd raised her brow. "But you have two boys already. Are you sure you want another?" Between the lines, she was expressing more the concern about our ages and the expense of another child than examining the why. *Haven't you had enough work with these two children?* she implied. *Moreover, aren't they enough?*

Anyway, that's what I heard in her questions. She was ultimately supportive of our choice, but I couldn't help but feel I should be happy with what we had. After all, by virtue of my relationship with Rebecca, I'd had two little boys, and I hadn't had to go through the pregnancy or the early developmental years with them.

But that was precisely what I missed.

When I first got up the nerve to take my mother to lunch and explain to her what we were doing, her reaction was simple: "Does Rebecca support this? Does she really want to do this?" And, "Well, if you want to put your body through this . . ."

She was referring more to becoming pregnant than the fertility treatments themselves. Pregnancy had been difficult for my mother, and it never seemed to give her warm fuzzies. I didn't know until my thirties that she had spent all her trimesters feeling sick and taking medication to help with nausea. But I did often feel, growing up, that children in general nauseated my mother, that they felt like an inconvenience, maybe a parasite. I was fortunate to hear the story of my own delivery, but it didn't help much. It was an emergency C-section. My mother was whisked away from my father, her glasses taken from her, leaving her virtually blind, the series of medications administered so she could feel nothing, numb to my emergence into the world. For both my parents it was a tale of great anxiety and separation, but one in which I ultimately prevailed. And they loved me, even though I also felt that I was their burden.

"My children are burdens," Rebecca once declared to her younger coworker, Stephanie. Stephanie was horrified, and she gasped.

"But it's true," Rebecca said. "Everyone is a burden. We are *all* burdens to each other."

This raised more indignation from Stephanie.

"It doesn't mean they are not worth it, Stephanie," she continued. "They are the greatest sources of my sorrow, but also of my joy. They're worth it every day."

Stephanie remained fixated on the negative connotation of that one word.

I understood the practical wisdom Rebecca conveyed. Each additional life on this planet is a life we all carry, even when we are not personally touched by it. We carry each other, and it can be an awesome load to bear. It can make us resentful, even furious, because we are individuals with egos, and we feel that with each additional person on the planet, our ego's survival is threatened.

Often, we have no choice as to whether another child is in our midst. We live with others' choices every day, just as much as we live with our own.

I thought about my Aunt Eileen, the way the car accident that occurred when she was eleven years old had affected her, pushing her into a coma from which she awoke and had to learn everything again, my middle-aged grandparents caring for their youngest child whose needs were beyond what they could handle, as had been the case even with their six other healthy children. The impact, the emptiness and grief from her accident, left traces throughout the family. My very Catholic grandmother admitted to me once that she had been planning on leaving my grandfather after her six older children had grown and just before Eileen's accident. She was closer and more resolved than she'd ever been to changing her life; and then Eileen was hit by a car on her way across the street to the ice cream truck.

Grams would say "God had other plans," or "It was a blessing in disguise, I guess, because it brought Grandpa and I closer together again." I couldn't help but wonder about the life she could have had instead, or the life Eileen might have had.

As the first grandchild on that side of the family, born four years after this accident, I was acutely aware of the loss of many dreams that stemmed from Eileen's disaster and, later, her handicaps. I also understood what it meant to be a burden to others. Even though my grandparents cherished her, and her siblings did, too, whatever was tearing in the family's fabric before the accident became glossed over and buried below. I could see it in the way my Aunt Bea spoke to Eileen, frustrated by the traumatic brain injury that delayed her development. Bea often mimicked the condescension in my grandfather's tone and was far more prone to be short and irascible around Eileen, more disagreeable than she was with any of her family, except maybe Grandma. Others in the family seemed to follow Grandma's lead and speak to Eileen in a voice they reserved for fragile creatures, practically cooing at her. Both modes would aggravate me. I could see they were managing their guilt and anger in the best ways they could, but neither seemed to help Eileen grow up. She was burdened by the traumatic brain injury, but she was not dumb, and while she may have been stunted in her maturity and emotional understanding of the world, she was still growing and developing. I could see that. She needed encouragement and space to grow, nurturing that allowed her room to mature as capably as possible. Were they not seeing her? Would she always be stuck as the eleven-year-old chasing after her ice cream, even when she was thirty? I knew that children aged despite us, but do children grow because we let them develop into themselves, or do they stay stuck because we do not let them grow?

These thoughts plagued me at night when I was choosing to become pregnant. Not only did I worry about the additional burden of another mouth to feed on our moderate income, I worried about my responsibility as a citizen of the Earth, as a participant in life. Was it fair to knowingly add to the burden of a planet we had all contributed to damaging in some way? Was it fair to procreate when so many children who already exist are malnourished or neglected? What kind of future did this little one have to look forward to, and what could I do, what had I not yet done, to make it better?

When these thoughts overcame me, I'd think that I should step over my ego, my biological clock, and just press the Adopt button. That word gave me the shivers, too, because it was attached to the greater burden of money, so many dollar signs to invite one more life into our household, a life that had already been created and chosen, a human we would raise and love.

I hung onto the notion of the biological route because I wanted so desperately to know the experience of pregnancy, to carry this being inside me. I was less excited about labor, but knew in the end it would be worth it—I heard that said again and again, by so many women I knew. I hoped for the bond created by the pregnancy and the special time afterward. Sometimes I secretly fretted that it would feel different than my bond to Seth and Sawyer, different in a way that would somehow exclude them. I didn't want them to ever feel that way. I didn't want any divisiveness to exist between Rebecca, the boys, and me. We worked so hard to become a solid, peaceful, kind, and supportive family. I didn't want anything to destroy that.

And all the while, I was crazed with the desire to have this baby, even when I was turning us topsy-turvy. Even if it wasn't the best decision we could make, it was making itself for us.

I recalled my father's opinions about the *Steel Magnolias* movie, about the woman who jeopardized her health to have a baby. He thought it was an act of futility. He said it was stupid to do to herself and her loved ones. "All that just to have a baby? There are other things she could've done." It's true, I thought. As Rebecca would say, "There's always an element of selfishness in whatever we do, no matter how altruistic."

Then the summer day came when the doctor called me. He was not my usual doctor; he was an interim while my doctor was away. Unlike my doctor, he was much more anxious than sanguine. His voice rippled with urgency. "Ms. Majoya, we need to discuss this insemination that you're planning to have on Monday." I held my breath at the sound of his consternation. "You do realize that you will have to make a decision if this takes, yes? It is really important that you go into this fully aware of your options. You do realize that you have four fully ripened ova, and that there is a strong possibility this will lead to multiples, yes? Are you prepared to move forward, knowing the risks involved with multiple pregnancy? And I'm not saying you could not carry to term, but that you do have a possibility of quadruplets, and this often has other ramifications." I knew enough about fertility treatments to recognize that multiples were a possibility. Rebecca would respond enthusiastically to the notion of twins. "Built-in playmates," she'd assert, while the idea of a singleton overwhelmed her more. From her experience, she knew how to handle two children at once, but one child—who would play with it all the time?

"I understand there are risks," I told him.

"But do you truly realize the risks?"

His accent, slightly Indian mixed with a bit of Brooklyn dialect, was drawn out more with his concern. "You do realize that, often with this kind of multiple pregnancy, you would be looking at terminating at least one of the fetuses for the health of everyone. And we can't always produce perfect results. You may not have a healthier fetus make it through this. It is an incredible process with anticipated burdens."

There was that word again.

"You do not have to go forward. If you would prefer, we can hold off until a future month."

"I need to talk it through with my partner."

"Of course you do, by all means. Please call me with your decision."

I wished my choice rested on his shoulders.

Could we risk this? Would we?

I was reminded of our friend Susan, who'd told us about the excruciating process with her daughter after she became pregnant with multiples as a result of fertility treatments. Susan had been there for her daughter when they placed the needle into the amniotic sac and determined that one of the three fetuses would be destroyed. Susan teared up as she relayed the pain it caused them. She expressed deep concern about the risks of twins, even, and pointed to the issues her daughter's children faced, with one child coping with a series of health problems even as the other thrived.

"You know," she'd said, "in the case of twins, often one is healthier—more robust—than the other."

The thought of twins did not overwhelm me. Even in high school I used to think that I had a strong possibility of having twins. I knew they were somewhere in my maternal family history, and I felt, much like I thought I was a Fertile Myrtle, that they were a likely reality.

The reality of twins was a different story, though. I knew friends who had hallucinations with twin infants because of sleep deprivation and the lack of available people to share the burden with. It would be quite a toll on us, on our current sense of comfort. Rebecca affirmed a blessing in the joy each child brought with them. But I knew she wasn't forgetting, unless momentarily, the endless nights with a colicky baby, the incessant needs of little ones—needs that could never be fully met, only met as best as possible at the time.

And yet, despite my better judgment and the doctor's refrain when I called him back, despite all that, we chose to take the risk.

Some part of me already knew it was a calculated one and that the quadruplets-to-be would never manifest, so there was little to multiply with.

But there was, of course, because we still had the boys.

They were quickly growing into men, their voices deepening, their inches adding up alongside them on the measurement chart we'd handwritten on the doorjamb of the kitchen. All that testosterone. All that newfound sexuality. All that potential fertility.

Some part of me felt like I was racing time against them. It would only be a matter of years, of months, before they were holding their own babies in their arms. I felt foolish, then, about being resentful of their likely procreative abilities, much as I thought about Rebecca's sister and her seemingly never-ending addition of children, year after year.

If I felt they were my boys, really, then how could I not rejoice in the prospect of a healthy grandchild? But it was often those times when I felt younger than my physical age and when the eleven-year gap between Rebecca and me expanded. I was not ready to be anyone's grandmother. Heck, I was just trying to have our baby and, in my mind, grandmothers were at least fifty years old, and I was still in my midthirties. I had family members who were just getting started with kids at my age. The people who were grandmas already, well, they'd had babies in their teens. And I'd never have been one of *those girls*.

But wait a minute. I *was* one of those girls by virtue of agreeing to parent Sawyer and Seth. I would have been seventeen and nineteen if I'd given birth to them. It didn't seem possible. It was as if I'd been living somebody else's life all these years. But the reality was that it was me in there all along. And didn't I know, didn't I feel that they were our boys? Or was it that they were more *like* my boys?

"If I raised them, they'd have been like my boys," I once heard a woman at work say to me when describing her stepsons. But I did help raise them, didn't I? I mean, I *thought* I was there. I tried to create a conscious love with Rebecca. Didn't I also do that with them?

I vacillated between feeling very close to them and feeling distant. I didn't want to have a push-me-pull-you kind of agreement with them, but might I have done that, trying so hard to maintain emotional distance and give them space so they would not be overcrowded by too many helicopter parents? Then again, I didn't want them to think I was as remote and unavailable as I felt many of the adults in my life were. How is it that I tried to behave differently from my parents, only to realize I was replicating similar patterns?

Hearts can be vastly overlooked—just consider the heart dis-ease of our world. I didn't want it to be a little too little, a little too late for my heart, or for others', but I had not remembered it is a muscle. It strengthens when we use it and weakens when we close off the passageways to it. Does love do this as well? Or does it thrive regardless of whether we nourish it? I suppose that is exactly what our burdens are here to teach us, whether we learn this or not.

LABOR PAINS
Rebecca, 2014

"She's at the hospital, her water broke!" I screech at Sallyann as she is coming out of the bathroom from showering.

"What?" she looks bewildered.

"Our lawyer just called. She said that Delilah called her lawyer to tell her to tell us that she is in the hospital." I try to slow down a bit, without much success. "She and Corey are at the hospital, her water broke last night, and she has been there since early this morning."

"We just saw them yesterday. I thought she wasn't very dilated." Sallyann, still wrapped in a towel, looks at me, perplexed. "What do we do?"

"We go! Delilah told us yesterday she wanted us there for the birth. She contacted her lawyer to get us there. So . . . let's go." I am trying hard to be calm and it isn't working. It might as well have been my water that busted all over the floor. "Call work, let them know you're not coming. I'll grab some clothes . . ."

"Clothes?" Sallyann is looking at me like I have three heads. The way I am all over the place, I probably look like I do.

"In case we are there overnight. We probably will be."

We thought we had another week, but this baby boy was ready to make his entrance. One thing about babies— they have their own timetable. After waiting more than eight years, it is impossible to wrap my brain around the fact that we are in labor!

Pulling into the parking lot of the small hospital, we easily find a parking spot near the entrance. All three babies I will raise, all born at the same hospital— strange to believe. One of the reasons we chose not to go through DCF in our city was that I didn't trust the privacy. I had worked with the population here for almost twenty-five years as a social services provider. I couldn't go into a grocery store without bumping into someone I had helped along the way. With such a small population, coupled with the high number of people in poverty or experiencing a crisis at some point in their lives, I knew pretty much everyone by sight, even if not by their name. I had not wanted to get involved with a child from this town and then figure out what to do when I saw them at the creemie stand every summer. Yet here we are, where I never thought we'd be.

We know which floor to go to and even what direction to head down the hall. It is the same area I had been in for recovery from my hysterectomy ten years ago. I had visited countless mothers and friends here when they had births and other gynecological surgeries over the years. Having been here so much, I knew a couple of the nurses, along with the low number of opportunities for nurses living in the area. This was the only hospital for forty miles.

At the nurse's station, I hesitate only a moment.

"We are the adoptive parents for Delilah Miller's baby," I announce. "Can we see her?"

"Great to meet you both." The nurse comes around the desk to shake our hands. "Delilah told us you two would be coming. Let me see what is going on in her room first, okay?"

"Of course." I step aside as she heads down the hallway.

She is quickly back out of the room she'd disappeared into.

"The doctor is in with her now. You can wait in this room for families." She gestures toward a room with a TV on the wall and eight padded chairs, two of which are filled.

Debbie, Delilah's mother, is not happy to see us—that's obvious. No matter what she had said about supporting her daughter's decision, the cold greeting tells another story.

"Hi there." We both greet Debbie as warmly as we can muster.

"Hi," she says, barely looking up from her cell phone.

She is texting forcefully, as if her life depended on it.

We greet the person next to her, sitting cross-legged on the chair. She is younger than Debbie, thin and lithe. She reaches out to shake our hands, meeting our eyes.

"Hi, I'm Mira. Or they call me Mimi, my sisters do," she says calmly. *Could this person be from the same family?* I wonder.

"I am Debbie's younger sister and kind of a sister to Delilah, since we are close in age. So, you are the couple who are adopting her son?" she asks innocently.

I am taken aback by her calling the baby Delilah's son. Delilah never refers to the baby like that. She says *the baby* or even uses the term *it* nonchalantly when talking to us about the child she's carried. The child she is in labor with. The one we would be taking home as our son.

"Yes." Thankfully, Sallyann is not thrown, like me. She is courteous and engages with Mira while taking a seat. I sit next to Sallyann, across from Debbie and Mira. We are not, thank goodness, directly facing the TV as the two of them are. I find it so distracting.

"I am pregnant too," Mira says eagerly.

"Yeah, so I'll have one baby to hold," Debbie interjects, never lifting her eyes from the phone. She gets up and heads out the door. "Gotta find the bathroom," she says to no one in particular as she leaves.

"Never mind her," Mira says quietly, as if Debbie might hear from the bathroom down the hall. "She gets this way. She'll be fine."

I am not sure what fine would look like. I look forward to seeing it, though.

Mira continues to talk about choices for her birth; she is due in March and can hardly wait.

"I plan to breastfeed, of course, and I have toys picked out that are made from natural products." She is obviously what Vermonters call "granola."

When Debbie comes back from the bathroom, the nurse follows her into our little space.

"The doctor has gone if you want to go see Delilah now," she says brightly, gesturing toward the hallway.

"Which room is it?" I ask.

"Four," Debbie says as she walks by us and down the hall without looking toward us.

Sallyann and I pause. Once the two of them are gone we look at each other, perplexed.

"Do we go or stay here?" I ask her.

"Your guess is as good as mine," she responds.

"Well, I think Delilah should know we came as soon as we knew. We don't want her to think we aren't interested," Sallyann says.

"Good thinking. Then I'll go get coffee." I smile.

Delilah looks up at us and gives a small smile as we enter. Corey sits, leaning against her on the bed. He watches over her shoulder as she texts. The two chairs in the room are filled with her mother and Mira, so we move awkwardly to her bedside.

"Good morning," I offer cheerfully.

"Morning," she says softly in return.

"We wanted you to know we came as soon as the lawyer called us," Sallyann says gently. "Can we get you anything?"

"She can't eat, and that's making her cranky," Corey says, giggling a little.

"Well, do you want anything, Corey?" I offer.

"I would love a coffee," he says eagerly.

No surprise, since he was quite the coffee drinker when we had met previously.

"Sure," I say. "I need some, too. Lots of cream and sugar?" I knew already he liked it sweet.

"Yes." He seems pleased we remembered his preference.

We leave the room, happy to have a purpose and glad to be out of the cramped space with its discomforting company.

By 2 p.m., we have been in and out of the room twice to see if Delilah needs anything or if we can support her in any way. Corey has had two large coffees so far, and we took him down for a big breakfast at noon. It is crowded with Debbie and Mira in there. All of them, including Delilah, are on their phones every minute, so there is little conversation. They also have the TV on constantly, with the volume up. We sit in the waiting area or go to the cafeteria for food.

Debbie and Mira join us in the waiting area.

"Hi, there," I greet them. "Is everything okay?"

"The doctor is back again. I hope he does something to hurry this along," Debbie reports.

"I don't think it is a good idea to use forceful methods," Mira adds. "I plan to have my birth as natural as I can. No drugs."

"Humph. We'll see," Debbie states while typing on her phone.

We mindlessly look at the TV for about fifteen minutes, then the nurse appears.

"You can come back in now," she offers. "The doctor has ordered Pitocin, since Delilah isn't dilating."

"Thank goodness," Debbie says as she gets up. "I'm going to have to get Eloisa soon"—referring to her younger daughter. "Let's get this show on the road." She heads back to the room.

Mira rolls her eyes and follows.

A few minutes later Mira appears to say goodbye to us on her way out.

"I have to get home now. Things to do, you know. Nice to meet you both." She shakes our hands and smiles as she goes. A few minutes later we see Debbie walk by.

"Should we go back to the room?" I ask Sallyann.

"No idea," she replies, and we laugh nervously.

We had been talking, texting, and trying to stay calm, but it is getting exhausting. We decide to go and check in on Delilah. With the Pitocin in action, she is visibly uncomfortable.

"How are you?" I ask tentatively.

"Okay," she says, but I am not convinced.

"Do you want us to get you ice chips or water?" I ask.

She points to the nightstand, which holds a cup of both items.

"I guess you are set then." Sallyann nods.

Delilah forces a half-smile. She squeezes Corey's hand as a contraction hits hard.

When it recedes she says softly, "I just want some

KFC." We smile and assure her she will get some as soon as she can eat. We slip back out the door to the waiting area.

About a half hour later we have the pleasure of meeting Eloisa. She enters the waiting room exuberantly, with the energy of a child with more caffeine in her diet than vegetables. She is bouncing and asking questions of Debbie that are completely ignored.

"Mommy, where is Delilah?" Eloisa inquires. "When do we get to see her? When will she have the baby? Are we going to eat now?" The last question does get answered.

"Yes," Debbie says impatiently. "Just let me get set down and I will open the bags."

The McDonald's bag is opened and Eloisa is quick to dive into it.

"As soon as we're done, we'll go in. We don't want to eat in front of Delilah; she can't eat," Debbie tells Eloisa.

I am glad she is thoughtful about the food.

"Maybe we should go get dinner," I say to Sallyann. We head back to the cafeteria, where we can also avoid any chaos in the waiting area.

As we walk past the nurses' station one of them motions us over.

"I wanted to catch up with you two. I just got permission to give you a room." She smiles. "My name is Maddie. I am on for the night."

"A room?" Sallyann questions.

"Oh yes." Maddie smiles. "You get a space of your own, as the adoptive parents. As soon as the baby comes, as long as he is healthy, he will be taken to the room with you," she explains. "Delilah made it clear to us and the hospital social worker that she does not want to see the baby. So we will bring him right in to you so you can bond with him."

Sallyann lights up, and so do I.

"Besides," she says more quietly, even though no one is within earshot, "it looks like you could use some privacy."

KENDALL AND DCF
Rebecca, 2013

"Can you be with my son at the hospital?" My friend Mary's voice was alarmed. Her life was rarely calm, but she sounded stressed, even by her standards.

"Yes, I think so. I can check with Sallyann. Why, what is going on?"

I am thinking about the last time we met this strawberry blonde friend of ours at the hospital. Sallyann had played the harp for her son, who had head trauma and back injuries from a motorcycle accident. Mary has five sons with three different fathers from three very different phases of her life. A life that has been long and held little mercy for her, or her sons.

"It's Chad. His ex-girlfriend had the baby. She had dirty urine going in, before the birth, but it still sounds like they will let the baby go home with her. He doesn't think he can advocate for himself. With his brain injury, he doesn't feel like he is a good choice. Maybe they will let you have her."

"Let us have her?"

"Yes, it's called unrelated kinship care. You know our family; you are as good as next of kin. You and Sallyann could have her. I know you've been wanting a baby."

It began to sink in. She wanted us to have this baby, the tiny baby girl . . . newborn.

Mary knew we had been trying to have a baby, trying to acquire a baby for so long. She didn't believe this was Chad's daughter . . . but she didn't know, not for sure. I knew the mother was using drugs, at least heroin; this was not small potatoes for potential developmental issues.

"But, your granddaughter?"

"*No*. No, no, no, I don't think it is really Chad's. After his accident, he was told he couldn't have children. He says he used condoms anyways, and I mean, he couldn't trust who she had been with. It could be many different fathers, but not Chad. We know she only told him that to get money from him. He is the only one of the bunch of guys she's been with who has any money."

"But does he want her?" I was shaking a bit, inside and out.

"For now . . . but like I said, she can't be his. He won't want her if she isn't his, I am sure of that." Mary sounded convinced.

He won't want her? My heart wanted to believe Mary. I was not sure how to explain this to Sallyann. She had known about Chad's girlfriend being pregnant but not these other details. I felt hope and anxiety, and what else?

I didn't know how to describe it. A twist of emotions that are so difficult to sort, to be named.

We arrived at the hospital at around 11 a.m. The baby was asleep on Chad's chest. He had his arms around her tenderly. He kissed her head as we entered. Whether or not he was the father, he certainly was bonded already to this tiny thing, swimming in premature clothes at just under five pounds.

We tiptoed in and peeked at her, and he asked if we wanted to hold her.

"Of course." Sallyann was quick to respond. She picked up the little bundle and held her close as her lamblike cries filled the room.

The doctor briskly entered and asked for her to be put into the bassinet to be weighed and checked for withdrawal symptoms.

We found out that, over the last few months, Britt, the birth mom, had been on Suboxone, which a baby must withdraw from. The mom had not always been reliable to avoid heroin either. The baby's little arms were stiff, and she shook when the doctor pulled her up by her arms.

Britt came out of the bathroom, cell phone in hand, texting furiously.

"I'm going out for a cigarette," she said in Chad's direction, taking no notice of the doctor with the baby.

After the check-in, the doctor left the room, the baby still in the bassinet.

Sallyann picked her back up. "What is her name, Chad?"

"Kendall. Her older brother named her."

"Kendall. That reminds me of Kenzie, the nickname for our niece Mackenzie," she said as she looked directly at me.

"Yeah, it's a cute name for a cutie." He was enamored of her. I could not imagine him giving her up easily, as Mary seemed to think he would.

Mary entered the room with bags, all blustering.

"Here you are, Chad. I found two more preemie-size sleepers at JCPenney. You would think in a town where seven out of ten babies are born addicted to opiates there would be more preemie clothes," Mary proclaimed.

"Maybe that is why they don't have them," I answered her. "They are sold out, not that they don't stock them."

She fussed over the baby in Sallyann's arms.

"Kendall looks happy there." She winked at me.

"So, how soon will they do a DNA test, Mary?" I asked, trying not to sound as anxious as I was to know if it was Chad's child, her grandchild.

"As soon as we are out of here, we are going to court to get an order for one," she responded enthusiastically. "Britt can't wait to ask for money from Chad, since he's on SSDI. She knows his child will get a paycheck, and she wants it."

"So, she won't fight you on a DNA test?" I asked.

"Oh no. She wants it. Right, Chad?" Mary said.

"I guess so." He shrugged.

He didn't seem as eager to believe ill of Britt. I could see in his eyes the longing for a family. No one had thought that would be possible after the motorcycle accident—the severe head injury, neck broken near the skull—that could have killed him. It was amazing he wasn't paralyzed.

"You would be happy with the girls raising Kendall, right Chad?"

I was horrified that she was so being blunt about this as he took the baby back from Sallyann and kissed her head.

"Well, yeah. Then I could see her, and I can't really raise her, with my bad memory."

"But you would want to?" I was not sure I was understanding him or their intentions.

Mary redirected the conversation by opening the bag of new clothes and making a fuss over them.

"Look at this one, Chad. Don't you love the little bunnies on it?"

"Aw, that is cute, Mom." He smiled.

He couldn't do it, he just couldn't raise a baby on his own, and how would the court allow a twenty-four-year-old with a severe head injury and a felony record have a baby that wasn't his?

We had a chance; I believed it. We had a chance to have this tiny baby girl.

Sallyann had met Mary at a gathering at my place. I'd invited friends I knew would come. I didn't want to deal with an empty room after cooking up treats and expecting to be surrounded by women who had been a part of my thirty-seven-year history and were trustworthy to do what they said they would.

I was excited to introduce Sallyann to my friends and to enjoy some wine and relaxed fun together. Mary was immediately keen on doing tea leaf readings for us all. She had learned from her grandmother, who was more like a mother to her than her mother was. Each person coming through the door brought a teacup that was special for a multitude of reasons. Mine was a gift from my mother, my very first teacup. It was small, holding only six ounces, and had carousel horses all around it, as if freed from the carousel and now forever flying in circles. It was supposed to work better if it was a special cup, according to Mary.

The small living room was filled with twelve women sitting in soft chairs, on the love seat, on kitchen chairs, and on the floor. Wine and tea were abundant and so was the laughter—of women who'd known each other for years, and others just getting acquainted.

Sallyann and I sat on the floor next to each other. I'd occasionally get up to refill food trays and greet new people coming to the door.

Mary passed out loose tea in several varieties, dropping a generous tablespoon into each cup. The water boiled and was poured onto the expectant leaves; we awaited our destinies.

"You will be getting a large package soon," Mary exclaimed over my cup.

"What kind of package?" I inquired, amazed that this was somehow displayed in the leaves, now sloshed around the edge of my near-empty cup.

"It could be many things, really," Mary replied.

"It could be a person, money, a literal package in the mail. Something new will arrive in your future. It could come in many different ways. A raise, a gift, a new person in your life." This made me look at Sallyann, but she was already here. Did that count? I wanted her to be a permanent part of my life, so it was easy to hope that this would be the reference point. I had known her only a couple of months, but I loved her so dearly. It was as if we had been together for so much longer, perhaps lifetimes . . . Mary wouldn't argue with this. I had been the skeptic about past lives, but not since I met Sallyann. She had changed my life, and I believed she would continue to.

We returned to the hospital the next day with our own teeny preemie outfits we'd found at a secondhand store. We had taken Sallyann's mom along, and we had all oohed and aahed over the teeny-tiny clothes. They were planning to release the baby and Britt. We had made phone calls yesterday to the Department of Children and Families requesting to be earmarked as a kinship care option for Kendall if it was deemed unsafe for her to go home with her mom. The caseworker we met was psyched to have anyone who might be interested in giving a baby a home, and made a plan to do a preliminary home visit in a few days. She hinted that there were lots of other babies if this didn't pan out the way we thought it might.

Chad was still there, Kendall asleep on him, when we

quietly peeked in. He motioned us forward.

"You can take her." He gestured willingly; Sallyann didn't hesitate.

"We brought some clothes we found that are tiny," I said. He admired the little bunnies and the moose on the sleepers.

"Where is Britt?" I asked.

"Out for a cigarette." Just as he said it, she appeared.

"I can't wait to get out of here," she stated briskly and climbed into the bed, tucking covers around her. She seemed to take no notice of her baby in Sallyann's arms.

The doctor came in and asked Britt if we were family.

"No, but it's fine, you can talk with them here."

He read off the most recent tests of the baby and of Britt's urine.

"So, it looks like you can be discharged today with your baby."

"She can take her home?" Chad asked incredulously.

"Yes, everything is okay. She needs to bring her to the pediatrician in two days," he stated matter-of-factly, and walked out.

"Thank god!" Britt exclaimed. She reached out toward Kendall and said, "Let me change her diaper so we'll be ready."

As Britt put her on the bed, her phone rang. Picking it up and tucking it under her chin, she talked while taking off Kendall's little onesie and diaper. Kendall cried. Her tiny sounds came in little bursts.

"What do you mean?" She spoke into the phone, stopping with the baby-changing and giving all her attention to the conversation. The baby continued crying, completely naked. Her little arms stiff, pulled in at her sides.

I could see Sallyann's stress and I felt it in my soul. This was not good, not a sign that the doctor had any intention of the little one going with us. She was free to go home with Britt. Even though, just four days ago, she pissed urine with heroin in it . . . now she could take home this child—her child.

The intense scrutiny that we had undergone overwhelmed me. I thought of the fingerprinting, the references, the background and motor vehicle-history checks we had paid for, the multitude of questions, the interviews and visits with the adoption agency. The weeks at the foster care classes. My eyes met Sallyann's and the pain was evident. I went out to the hall and saw the doctor with a nurse, talking about another patient. I went up to them, and the doctor brushed by, heading into another room. I asked the nurse, "Is there any reason the baby isn't going to foster care? I mean, the mom's urine . . ."

"Britt is fine. No one has brought her anything. She's been clean since the birth." She walked away.

My heart was crying; could everyone hear it? It seemed so loud.

I made my way back to the room. Sallyann was holding the now re-clad Kendall in her arms, and Britt was dressed, eager to get out where she could smoke more easily.

Chad seemed bewildered but was smiling. Britt's phone rang again and she said she'd be right down. A woman came in with a wheelchair. Britt got in. The baby was eased out of Sallyann's arms and into hers.

We all gathered bags and purses; we headed to the elevator. At the first level, it was a short walk to the door where Britt's mom waited impatiently in the car.

"The car seat is in the back," she said, barely noting the baby.

Kendall was fastened in, and then they drove off.

"Do you need a ride, Chad?" I asked, knowing he could not drive due to his head injury.

"No, my brother is on his way now," he said. All three of us were in a befuddled state.

We hugged him goodbye, asked him to call if he needed anything. Then we walked to our car. It seemed miles away, but it was only a couple hundred feet from the door.

It was over. It was all over. The DCF worker would still pay us a visit, but there would be no need. We were back to the beginning.

GIMME THE BABY
Rebecca, 2014

"Gimme the baby," we would whisper to each other when we saw infants in a store or on the street.

"Gimme the baby." Then giggle a nervous laugh that came to diffuse the fear that there would never be a tiny little one in our arms, even though one had grown in our hearts for years. Years that kept adding up, full of failed attempts at having the pile of diapers and tiny clothes in our room, filled with the new smell of a little life, that glorious fragrance of a newborn baby.

Everywhere we went we seemed to run into young mothers pushing strollers with two or three babies in them. Cell phones in hand, lit cigarettes dangling, thoughts obviously elsewhere, they meandered along, apparently oblivious to how favored they were to be able to produce those precious little ones. No wonder we felt like saying:

Give us the baby.

Give us the baby to hold and read to and care for.

We didn't make a lot of money but we had a lot of love to give, so why should only those with lots of money, or lots of fertility, be the ones to get the babies?

Gimme the baby. Just give him to us, and we will hold

him and diaper him and take him for vaccinations on schedule.

I wanted to fill the world with my rage, in hopes that somehow the universe would change so we could create a tiny being that looked like us, had our mix of traits. But, for the time being, that was impossible.

The knock at the door startled us even though we were waiting for it, waiting to do our adoption home study. We had filled out over forty pages of information. Each of us had separately answered all the regular questions found on a work application, such as employment history, education, references, and hobbies. Then there were all the pages of questions about the child. How would we raise a child as far as parenting tactics, and what kind of philosophy did we have around child-rearing? What nationalities were okay, what mixes of races, and how would we address a child's cultural needs if their culture is different from ours? Then, of course, we had to relay the information about our own upbringings. What are our personal histories, do we have siblings, and where were we raised? What could be left for the home visit that is supposed to take three hours, one hour with each of us separately and an hour together?

Emma is kind in demeanor and soft-spoken, as she has been for every other meeting we've had. We offered her tea before Sallyann stepped out of the room so the two of us, Emma and I, could complete our portion of the interview.

"You have a lovely home here," she said with warmth and authenticity.

I was anxious, but of nothing in particular.

"How long have you lived in this house?" she asked, sipping her tea, still quite hot.

"Thirteen years," I answer. "All of our life together. We tried to have a baby for the past seven years using donor sperm with Sallyann, but no luck. I had a partial hysterectomy, you probably already saw in my paperwork," I said, not sure how much to say or if I was talking too much.

"That's right," she said writing notes on her yellow legal pad. "How are you feeling about releasing the idea of the baby having any of either of your genetics?" She looked at me when speaking even though she had a thick printed-out pile I assumed were the questions she had to cover. She had been at this for years.

"I am sad, but it certainly isn't a deal breaker for me." I immediately wondered if that was a good enough answer. How could I know?

"Of course, or we wouldn't be here today." She smiled and jotted notes.

The questions went on for over an hour, especially with the questions about each member of my family. I explained how my elder brother had died of brain cancer, and answered several questions about each of my three sisters and my parents.

"How often do you speak with her?" she asked, of my youngest sister.

"Not often, although we do text sometimes," I responded. "She has eight children and is not planning on stopping, as far as I know."

"Eight, wow, she has a big family. Are they all birth children?" she asked casually.

Of course she asked, I thought. No one else ever has asked that question in regard to her kids, but of course Emma would not assume they were all her natural-born kids.

"So, do you have any friends or family who have adopted?" she asked when we were done with the details of my relationships with each member of my family of origin.

"Yes," I responded, and went on to explain about my first cousins, and friends who have adopted, and how they were all welcomed as family.

Sallyann came downstairs from our bedroom to go to the bathroom and, to my relief, Emma stated she was about ready for her. I would never have believed that Emma could have over an hour and a half of questions for me, but she did.

Sallyann exited the bathroom and warmed Emma's tea, and I headed upstairs to our bedroom to give her privacy. Well, that was the premise. I was just glad to be off the hot seat. Some of the questions were similar to those on the questionnaire, but so much harder to answer in person. To write down that my parents had used corporal punishment was one thing, or that my brother had molested me. When a pair of eyes were looking into your soul and determining by each word that comes out of your mouth if you are a fit parent, that is entirely different.

I lay there and thought about the boys. Sawyer was almost done with college, and Seth was headed off on his own next month. How did we do? Should we have another child?

How could I be asking this after all we have already been through? The IVF, the donors, the foster care classes; I do want another child.

I thought about her question with regard to disabilities. I did not feel capable of dealing with large-scale medical issues, but so many others are undetectable. If they were detectable, would I care? Some considered autism a deal breaker, but Seth was a joy beyond imagining. No one I can think of loves as unconditionally as that kid—young man, I corrected myself. It was all such a crapshoot anyway, no matter whose genes were involved. Even after we are born anything can happen to change who we are. We can get an illness that affects us physically or mentally. My second cousin was in an accident at age twenty-one. He had been on his own, working, living with a girlfriend, and bam! A truck hit him and he was in the hospital, rehab for almost a year, and then living with his parents again, in a wheelchair. He would never think as clearly or talk as well as before. He would always need help.

Once we said yes to another human being in our lives, it would be *yes* for us. We would hold and cherish this little being forever. Whatever is and whatever will be. No backsies. Just please . . . *gimme the baby.*

We are at the will of others, another to decide that we are the arms that should hold the baby. Another mother will have to choose us, to connect to us through photos, to read the booklet we have painstakingly put together. Somehow she will decide from that, without seeing into our hearts.

Much as we had hoped with the sperm donors, another mother will hope we are telling the truth of our lives, that the pictures are truly reflective of a joyful place where someone else will raise her infant to an adult.

Again, we are completely at another woman's mercy.

Please, please be merciful . . . this time.

PART TWO

That fall is the release, the consummation

BIRD AND BIRD
Sallyann, 1985

Birds of a feather flock together, or so they say. Mom and Dad and I got more than we bargained for with those yellow finches. After the squeaky-toy chirps of the little bird fluttering up to her nest, we kept waiting. Then one day, Dad opened their cage, and we saw it.

An egg, no bigger than my little toe, so miniature it made my ten-year-old fingernails look humongous by comparison. It was a pale blue iridescent color, somewhat matte, no sheen like the store-bought chicken eggs in the refrigerator.

I squealed at the sight of that smallness. Like so many children, all small-scale things were designated as magically cute, subsumed under the world of dollhouses and books like *The Littles*. And in the world of kid-dom, tiny objects made me feel as gargantuan as the adults in my life seemed to be.

I watched the little birds hopping back and forth on their perches, whizzing to and fro in a flurry of activity from the plastic water dish to the plastic seed dish. It wasn't so long before that my dad and I had traipsed into the pet store of the Cherry Hill Mall in search of a Christmas gift for my mom. I adored Christmas shopping with Dad. It was the only time of the year that he seemed willing to shop without grumbling, and I'd see his eyes twinkle merrily, reflecting the seasonal sparkle of lights strung everywhere. It was also the time we would go together and pick out gifts special for my mother, and he seemed not just happy to do it, but overflowing with the generosity of Santa.

I don't remember how he'd gotten it in his head that, in addition to some of the usual gifts we picked for her—a new nightgown, a new sweater, another special Hallmark ornament, a crystal doodad to add to her knickknack shelf—it was time to buy her some pets.

My allergies meant we could no longer have kitties, though I'd have done anything to bring one of those fuzzy little purrballs home. My mom was also fond of cats.

I wondered if she'd hinted to him that she'd like some birds. I knew she liked lovebirds. I thought that would be a fitting gift for her. Then Dad pointed to the little finches that were nearly the size of my fist.

Boy, did those creatures move and make noise! I loved their liveliness. I knew they could add some vivacity to our second-floor duplex.

I preferred the teal-toned finches, but Dad opted for finches in my least favorite color, yellow, because he thought the brightness would cheer my mom.

We picked up everything we needed: cage, seed, containers, and snacks, then asked the shop helper to find us a male and female.

With a male and female bird, we might have little finches!

Oh, I was so excited to imagine what that would look like.

I thought about the gray cat we had when I was six years old. She'd holed up in an undisturbed space in my bedroom behind my kitchen play set and gave birth to six miniature versions of herself. They came out as shiny little blobs of shrunken fur and squinty eyes, with dull tails. I was elated when I found them.

They were not what I'd imagined of newborn cats.

What could finches—so inky dinky—give birth to?

Turns out nothing.

Nothing but an egg.

"Dad, when will the egg hatch?"

"It needs to be incubated," he reminded me, as if I didn't know, "by Bird Number Two."

I was impatient. I wanted a date.

Mom never named them, but she was pleased when we brought them home. She flapped around the house like a larger version of her gift, excitedly putting all their items in the cage and looking for just the right place to set them up.

So I tried naming them something trite, like Romeo and Juliet.

Obviously, they were not supposed to be called by the same name if they were boy and girl, right? Nonetheless, we ended up referring to them as Bird and Bird. They were a unit, made somewhat anonymous but obvious by their names.

Bird Number Two refused to play along with the whole egg obsession. I grew frustrated with it. I would talk to it through the rungs of the cage that separated our worlds.

"Little bird, don't you know what you're supposed to do? Little bird, why won't you sit on top of that egg?"

It sat exposed in the little nest that Bird Number One had so carefully created from hairs, threads, and little pieces of twine and twigs my dad had laid on the bottom of the cage for it to retrieve.

"I think they gave us two girls," my dad announced one evening after I returned home from school, while Mom was in the kitchen cooking. The aroma of grilling hamburger wafted through the apartment. Dad said it with a smirk, as if he'd secretly hoped for that all along.

Mom responded from the kitchen, "But I thought you asked for a boy and a girl."

"We did," I replied indignantly, now feeling irked by the pet shop worker who *apparently* didn't know the genders of his birds, or failed to tell us otherwise.

I felt cheated.

No baby birds.

Just two *stinking* birds of the same sex. I knew my parents were fine with what we had.

They laughed it off. "I guess we have lesbian birds."

Now *my* feathers felt ruffled. In my little suburban

town, I did not think I knew any lesbians, but I'd heard the word used derisively on the school playgrounds. And in the mid-1980s the concept of gay was synonymous with that terrifying sexual disease, AIDS. It was touted everywhere, on the news, and in our Scholastic *Weekly Readers* at school.

Most of the same-sex messages I'd learned were subterranean, way worse than acquiring cooties. We didn't talk about it. We barely talked about people who lived *that lifestyle*, except when Mom would mention the one gay man who worked with her. He was an anomaly, somebody who was considered funny, but who never came to my house. As with pedophilia, it was the unspoken something you should just avoid. If it wasn't said, it wasn't real.

Did birds come that *way?* I wondered. Maybe they became lezzies on account of being stuck in a cage together without any guy birds. It made me chuckle to think that our birds were so off, little flapping oddities.

Why, they belonged in our home!

Two females in prison for life, within a metal-slatted space, with no chance of reproducing.

Bird and Bird, girl and girl.

Weird.

LABOR PAINS
Sallyann, 2014

A Series of Text Messages Sent to a Group of Family Members: October 22, 2014, 7:53 a.m.

SA: *Her water broke in the middle of the night! Her lawyer just called. We are on our way to the hospital now! Xoxo*

ERIN: *Oh my godddddd*

FRANNY: *You ok???*

SA: *Trying to breathe! She wants us in the delivery room!*

RACHELLE: *Love and light coming your way!!!!*

SA: *Thanks cuz!*

SETH: *OH MY GOD OH MY GOD YOU'RE GONNA BE THE BEST MOMS EVER!!!!!!!!!*

RACHELLE: *That's great!!!!!*

FRANNY: *Omg!!!*

FRANNY: *Yippeeee!!*

SA: *We love you, Seth! You and your brother*

have paved the way

SETH: *Text the second you know if it's healthy!*

Do you mind if I gush to my housemates about this?

How's the birth mom holding up?

Am I asking too many questions?

Should I shut up?

Ok I'm gonna shut up now.

But when you have time please answer the gush question first 'cause I wanna gush

IWANNAGUSH!!!!

Okay, shutting up

FRANNY: ☺ <3 ☺

SA: *Seth, you can gush all you want. It looks like it's going to be a slow process.*

JUSTIN: *Prayers and best wishes . . . love you!*

FRANNY: *So excited for you all! Hope to see you this weekend!!!*

I am extra conscious of Delilah, as if she is an attached limb. I keep trying to determine what she needs, and all she offers are monosyllabic answers. I notice she is even quieter when her mom is nearby, mostly interacting with Mimi and whispering things to Corey. Outside the room, the nurses ask us how it is going in there.

Ever since her little sister arrived, the space has become ignited with loud and boisterous energy. The nurses take notice.

"I think we'll go in shortly and check on Delilah, make sure she has some quiet time." The two nurses share a knowing glance.

There is nothing quiet about this day. It is a three-ring circus.

"Well," I say to Rebecca, "at least we know she has people to support her."

"Do you think anyone's really *present* to support her?" she asks.

The nurses have just told us they are preparing a room right around the corner from Delilah's, and I am anxious to get into our own space.

I don't know if Delilah wants us there, but Corey keeps affirming to us how much it means to both of them. It is such a balancing act of not intruding too much and still being available.

I feel like a relief pitcher, stepping in as needed, mostly trying to keep Corey calm. He is almost as jumpy as Delilah's six-year-old sister, constantly fidgeting, moving from space to space, hopping about in Tigger fashion.

Earlier in the day, his mom, Donna, stopped by between shifts at a local nursing assistant agency. Donna seems particularly concerned with Delilah's well-being. I can see she is trying to be kind to us as well.

"So, you're the adoptive parents?" she asks.

"Yes," we blurt out in unison.

"Well, that is a really special thing to do. I know that Delilah is ready to pop this baby out," Donna says emphatically.

I watch as Donna plops down in a seat across from

us, asking questions of Corey, fielding his excess energy. She seems sad, as if this is her biological grandbaby on the way and she isn't ready to see it go, but she is also a stoic and resolute woman.

If this is what the kids want, she would support them, I had no doubt.

Corey complains to her about the hospital, about the nurses. He is visibly anxious about the fact that Delilah's dilation is progressing slower than expected. He plunks down on his mother's lap like a four-year-old in need of comfort. It looks silly, almost like an elephant on top of a giraffe, although his wiry frame settles comfortably into the solidity of his mom's lap. *Is he really twenty-one?* I think, looking across the room at the two of them. At this moment, he certainly is not.

I watch Donna and Debbie's interaction, which is cordial. They don't have much to say, but then again who does, with Delilah's mom?

Debbie talks over Delilah as if she isn't in the room. As if Debbie is the one in labor who deserves the attention. Occasionally she addresses her daughter, but I wonder if she can hear the derisiveness in her voice. She is punitive. She wants Delilah to know she is irritated.

She also does not take Corey seriously, which vexes him to the core. Outside the room, he complains to us about how Delilah's mother or Mimi treat him.

"Mimi is such a know-it-all. She keeps telling us what to do and how to do it, just because she's into massage and other alternative medicines," he harrumphs.

I saw Corey say something, only to have Mimi laugh him off. His nostrils flared. I could see he wanted to punch Delilah's family members, but is expending whatever energy he has left over to try and control his behavior. Coffee and nicotine breaks are not cutting it.

The edginess in the room is palpable and I feel for Delilah, who is just trying to get through the day and to be considerate of the people surrounding her, not giving her a moment's peace.

But evidently, this is what she was used to.

We just want her to have a voice.

We want her to feel like we hear her above all the other noises, including our own.

Before we know it, in come more visitors. This time it is Corey's grandparents. Donna mentioned when she was here earlier that they wanted to come and wish Delilah the best, so she anticipated they would meet us.

Finally, we are escorted to our hospital room, practically a carbon copy of Delilah's, minus all the people. I joke with Rebecca. "Do you think we should move Delilah in here, maybe let everyone else hover in the other room?"

It is a breathing space, and I am so grateful to the nurses and hospital that they would provide us with one.

"Oh, no problem, honey," the nurse who'd been with us all day says as she enters the room with us. "It's actually quiet on the ward tonight, and it's important for the expecting parents to have their own space." She smiles at us.

I cannot get over the kindness with which the staff treats us.

"This is the room where we came to visit Zach after his first baby, remember?" I say to Rebecca. It is a small community, and hospital. We'd been there countless times for other people's new baby arrivals. I still can't believe that Zach, Sawyer's childhood friend, is now the father of two little ones. We often said he was like our other son. Our home felt like the home of my childhood best friend, Brooke; a place where all our friends could safely congregate. In our case, ours was the home where all our boys' friends felt welcome. This new baby on the way would be our third son but, in essence, we feel we've already had several other children. I remember one night our tenant waking us up to let us know a teenage Zach was asleep on our porch swing. We ushered him into the house, "What's going on?"

He said he had to get out of the chaos of his home, so he'd walked the seven miles to our house in the middle of the night. There was desperation in his eyes. "I just wanted a calm place to come," he said. "I hope you don't mind."

"Of course we don't, Zach," Rebecca said as she pulled up a chair for him in the kitchen. "You always have a home here."

Corey comes to the doorway of our new room, one of many visits he makes throughout the evening, especially as he grows ever more agitated and nervous about the labor.

"Hi," he says shyly, as he tacks his head around the door. "Can I come in?"

As we had with Zach, we welcome him. Already he feels like one of our boys. "My grandparents would like to meet you, if that's okay."

"Oh, how sweet," I say, and we get up to join them just outside the doorway.

They were salt-of-the-earth Vermonters. We know from Corey that Grandpa had his own business, which he tried to give Corey a chance at working in. Corey told us he wasn't successful, since working for his gramps was "too demanding." Gramps is tall. He has a commanding presence, but he is clearly not comfortable in social situations, especially awkward ones like this. That is okay, because his wife, short in stature with a rim of curly white hair, makes up for him. She is kind and empathetic, and I take to her instantly. She has a grandmotherly comfort about her.

She introduces the two of them, and Grandpa grunts when his name is said. Then she launches into a seemingly prepared speech about how wonderful it is to meet us. How much it means that we are willing to do this, that these kids have already spoken of how kind we are, what good parents we'll be. I can see she is also nervous but wants to assess us to make sure we are as decent as she's heard.

"Well, we don't want to take up too much of your time. We just wanted to meet you and to thank you. We wish you all the best with your new family."

I could have invited his grandma in for tea, if she'd have stayed. She is one of the most welcoming people we've been with all day, aside from the nurses. While it feels like Gramps has no idea what to do with a lesbian couple taking on a baby that was part of their family, though not biologically, he has the wherewithal to show up for the occasion. I give him credit for that, since he surely is much happier with his John Deere—or whatever he uses. Corey's family is genuinely concerned with the outcome for both Delilah and Corey. It comforts us to know that, after the birth, these young people will have some family who acknowledge them.

SAGE IS BORN
Rebecca, 2014

He is warm and soft and his head has the perfect smell of a newborn. Is there anything in the entire universe that smells this good? I have never seen Sallyann smile this way. Her whole being exudes joy, peace, and love. She was born for this, this holding of a newborn, holding our Sage. It is unreal. He is so tiny.

"Of course he is." She jests with me. "You just forgot how little the boys were."

"No, actually, they were never this little when I saw them, when I held them in my arms." Sage is a whole pound lighter than our youngest, well, our *old* youngest, was when he was born. Now we have a new youngest, and he is more welcome, I believe, than any baby who ever came to this planet, of any species, anywhere.

"Do you want to hold him?" Sallyann asks.

"No, not yet. He is so happy right there on your heart. Who wouldn't be?" I am wallowing in the wonder of our new family member.

They are skin to skin. He still has the film of baby wetness from the amniotic fluid. There truly is no purer baby smell on Earth.

The nurses have been beyond accommodating, giving

us our own room, right across from Delilah's, so we could have privacy and prepare ourselves for the birth.

"You need a place for your personal things, and a place we will bring the baby immediately, as long as it is healthy. Then you can bond as a family," the head of labor and delivery announced to us when we hesitantly appeared at her desk. It is odd for me to show up here without an extended belly. It is the same place I delivered both boys, about twenty years ago.

There is a fear in the pit of my stomach, but I ignore it. This time it is real. This time it is our baby.

I watched Delilah close her eyes tightly and turn her head toward Corey while she pushed, concentration and strength, bearing down to get this baby out of her uterus and out of her life. Now she can begin healing both body and soul, and move on from this unintended incident.

And we can begin what we have waited so long for. Over eight years—not just nine months—of anticipation are wrapped in our love as we embrace this little guy.

"Did you text the folks?" Sallyann asks softly.

"No, plenty of time for that later. This is just too precious," I respond.

His eyes are big and look at Sallyann with open, calm curiosity.

"Sage," Sallyann says to him gently. "Our little Sage-guy. Can you believe it? Here you are, and we are so in love with you. Yes, we are your mommies and we are so glad to see you." She sings a bit of a lullaby to him, swaying a little in the bed.

His little hand is caught on the string of the johnnie, and Sallyann looks at me, just a bit flustered.

"How do I untangle him without breaking his teeny fingers?" she asks me.

"He is amazingly flexible, thank goodness, or none of us would make it. By tomorrow this time, you will not worry about that anymore," I assure her.

I take his ring and middle finger and gently loosen them from her gown.

"Time for a washing!" I can tell the nurse is not eager to take him out of our arms. He had the second APGAR test while on Sallyann's chest. With seven of ten babies here born addicted to some substance, it is a delight to work with healthy babies. The nurses seem to appreciate our status, too. I'd been worried. So worried about being here, an outsider in the event so dear and so longed for. But, with the click of the machines, Sallyann in her johnnie, and the two of us, two moms, all feels right, as though all *is* right in the world.

"Can you believe it has been two hours since he was born, already?" I say, shocked.

"It seems life is on speed mode. How does that happen?" Sallyann takes her eyes off him briefly as she puts him safely into the nurse's capable hands.

"Here we go." The nurse swiftly and deftly washes him before us, then a quick check of all vitals under the warm light of the infant table. She rewraps him in blankets snugly, and looks back to us. We are mesmerized by her movements and his eyes and little wiggling limbs throughout the process. I reach out for him now.

"My turn." I smile and hold him to my breast, next to my heart. So warm, so sweet. "We are destined to be moms of little guys," I say to him, to his eyes searching my face. "You have more family you'll get to meet soon. You will like them, and they are going to love you, for sure. Two big brothers, what do you think of that?"

"Oh, that's not all, Sage. You are in a big Irish family. We hope you like lots of love and hugs," Sallyann croons.

"And great food and parties," I add. "It may be tough to learn to walk with all these people wanting to hold you."

My eyes meet Sallyann's. I sit on the bed next to her. "I think he is rooting. Do you want to put him to your breast?"

She turns toward the nurse, who gestures to go ahead. When Sallyann pulls back the johnnie, he snuggles in, and with just a bit of readjusting, he latches on.

"Wow," she exclaims. "That is a strong jaw for being so tiny."

We laugh; he pulls off and looks up at her face.

"I think he likes your laugh, mommy," the nurse adds.

Sallyann smiles. She is glowing. I can't imagine a better day in my life.

PART THREE

If I can take the dark with open eyes

ADOPTIVE MOM
Sallyann, 1992

I was in my usual post-lunch daze when I heard my Human Development teacher, Mrs. Hutchins, a formidable woman with large glasses and rosy cheeks, announce that we were going to have a special visitor, her former student, join us in class the next day to talk about a topic related to the chapter we were working on: adoption.

Adoption? Oh geez. What could we possibly discuss on that subject?

I was reminded of one of my childhood friends, Audrey, whose schoolteacher mom filled the walls of their home with Norman Rockwell paintings. Her dad towered over us in his police officer getup. To me, Audrey seemed to be the epitome of the "spoiled only child," whatever it was that made people wrinkle up their noses and look at me with apprehension—or jealousy—when they found out that I, too, was an only. Audrey had a spacious house and backyard, her own playroom, and any toy she ever wanted. She took dance lessons and played sports. She was pushed into the gifted and talented program, and made certain to remind our peers every chance she got, as if she thought this was a prerequisite for being a better person.

In high school, Audrey was still smart and performance-inclined, and also into drugs and sex with random guys. I'd heard that she was struggling with her lack of knowledge about her birth family, her roots. This confusion bled into everything about her and, for a person who seemed like she'd had the world at her feet, she behaved incredibly insecurely.

That's an adopted kid for ya, I guess, was pretty much how most of my friends and I judged her. Their moms give them up. They're unwanted. They don't know which way is up. Probably her mom had been crazy in just the same way that she was behaving.

We spoke this just as critically and arrogantly as she had behaved in elementary school, as if we somehow had our shit *so together* from the families we came from.

When I showed up for the class, I dropped my books and bags in the usual spot, but the room had been rearranged so our circular tables and chairs now faced the side wall, toward the chalkboard. Mrs. H. welcomed us more tenderly than usual, fussing over where we sat, inquiring why some of the class was not there on such an important day. I looked over at the classroom door, out the wall of windows, wishing for a way out. Such was my typical daily feeling in high school anyway, but the way the teacher was acting made the urge that much greater.

Then, to my surprise, Denise walked in.

Mrs. H. greeted her with an affectionate hug and

thanked her for joining us.

As our teacher was prattling on and introducing her to the class, I tried to recall the last time I'd seen Denise.

In my memory, she was standing on the school grounds with my friend Jessie, burning a cigarette down to the end, looking down her nose at us young'uns as we passed through the courtyard and in, through the reverberating bang of the metal doors.

Had it been since the spring of seventh grade?

What grade was she in then? Ninth?

I ran through a Rolodex of memories, filing one picture after another, as I tried to fill in the years between us.

Before us, Denise stood confidently. She was dressed like an adult, in professional attire, hair coifed stylishly. She looked out at her audience smartly.

Denise was in college now.

Although only a couple years away from me then, it seemed a world away as I looked at her. How was it that Denise appeared to be a different person from the one in my memory?

Did college do that for her?

Also, I realized I'd had no idea she was adopted. But then again, I didn't know much about her at all.

She began: "This is my story, and Mrs. Hutchins invited me in here to share this with you so that you have a better understanding of the choices that are out there." She leaned on that word, *choices*, as if it was imprinted in bold and she wanted us to see it.

Then Denise began to share how she'd gotten pregnant a few years before, while she was involved in a relationship she'd thought was "the love for me."

He quickly withdrew when she told him about her pregnancy.

She told us that she'd contemplated abortion but was just not comfortable with carrying that out. Somehow, in my presumptuous mind, I found that to be shocking. You mean someone like Denise wasn't a poster child for abortion?

Hmm. People really could amaze you.

Denise admitted she'd needed someone to turn to for help, and she was grateful that a few people in her life showed up when they did. She acknowledged Mrs. Hutchins at this point.

"I found out about an adoption agency," she said, "where I could have a voice in who my baby went with and know what happened to her."

The room was quiet, our rapt attention swirling around Denise as she described the stress and confusion of her pregnancy, the people she met through the agency—a loving husband and wife—who wanted her baby with all their hearts. She shared that she'd felt they were great parents who could provide her baby girl with so much more than she had the capacity to give at that time.

"I wasn't really sure what I wanted to do with my future, but I knew that I was not ready to be a parent, and I had some goals, like furthering my education."

She smiled broadly. "I do not regret my choice." Again, she leaned into that last word.

"Her parents send me letters and pictures regularly. We call each other on occasion, but mostly we stay connected through letters and photos. She is, to me, the most beautiful little girl. I am so proud of her, and I just know she has a far better future with her parents than I could've ever given her."

With this, she passed around photos of a little strawberry blonde, hazel-eyed girl, whose smile shined through her photo, making her joy appear three-dimensional.

I was teary-eyed. I looked over at Mrs. Hutchins, who was staring at Denise as proudly as if she were looking at her own daughter.

I felt deeply moved by Denise, by her selflessness and by her love for her daughter. I was impressed by her desire to give her daughter a grander life, as well as by her maturity in making that decision at sixteen, the same age as most of the people in the room, including me.

I was awed that she could share all this so openly with us, wearing her heart on her sleeve, no longer holding her hip out in defense.

Mostly, I realized I could never know how much any person held within, each of us a little egg of possibility, just awaiting incubation.

ANGIE'S VISIT
Rebecca, 2014

"Angie!" I am shocked to see the vice president of my board of directors from work at our hospital room door.

"I just had to go shopping; we haven't had time to arrange for a shower yet, but I had to see him. I'm just *so* excited for the two of you!" Angie is holding six paper shopping bags, and her large purse is slung over her shoulder. She plunks everything down on the chair near the window, smiling broadly, genuinely thrilled for us.

I give her a long hug.

"He is beautiful," she says over my shoulder to where Sallyann is on the bed, feeding him from a bottle.

"What is all of this?" I ask, gesturing to the bags I've taken from her. "Did the board drop off things to you for us?"

"Oh no, no, no. I just love babies! I am so excited for you both. Oh, what a little love. Oh my, look at that hair. Such a headful. Aren't you the sweetest thing?" She strokes Sage's hair and then pats Sallyann on the arm.

"Wow! That didn't take long, did it? You just started wanting to adopt in July, right?"

I often forget that most people are unaware of how long we tried fertility treatments, or that we had started the adoption trek over two years ago. It occurs to me how much and how little we can know about each other. Angie has been on the board for five years. I have known her for seven. Yet we keep so much to ourselves, so much hidden from one another. Angie has three little boys, adorable individuals, totally precocious. She leads the HR department at a large energy company and is a combination of tough, kind, and emotive joy. She could get more accomplished in an hour than most people could in a whole day.

"It's just amazing," is all I can say. "Hard to believe it is real."

When Sallyann lifts Sage to burp him, he lets out a great big one without even a pat on the back. We all giggle. "He is the best little burper," Sallyann exclaims.

"Of course he is!" Angie responds. "Can I hold him?"

"Yes, yes!" Sallyann says as she tightens the receiving blanket around him. "He might need changing soon, but yes, here you go." She deftly places him in Angie's outstretched arms. "He smells so good, so clean, and"— Angie inhales deeply—"just like a baby." Smiling from ear to ear, she sits in the soft chair at the side of the bed.

"Go on, now. Open the presents." She nods toward the bags.

"So, these are all from you?" I say, not knowing what else to say.

"Oh yes," she remarks casually. "Just a few things for the little man. Yes, aren't you a perfect little man, though," she exclaims as she rocks her body back and forth, gently kissing his head. "Did he sleep at all last night?"

"Yes," Sallyann replies eagerly. "He slept three hours,

ate well, and then three more. He slept tucked in our arms in bed. We just can't put him down."

"Of course you can't, and why would you?" I see that Angie has noticed the breast pump and accoutrements on the twin bed in our room. "Are you nursing?" She is incredulous.

"Yes. Well, I will be soon." Sallyann smiles, pleased that Angie noticed. "I am pumping every two hours and we ordered a kit so I can feed him on my breasts and he will get milk"—Googling on her phone as she speaks—"see the little tubes taped to the side of the breasts and the nipple? The formula is pulled from this container, hanging like a necklace."

Angie gets it immediately. "Ah, so when he breastfeeds, he is stimulating your nipples to produce and the formula will feed him in the meantime."

"Until my milk comes in, yes. Then I will be able to breastfeed." Sallyann is elated at the prospect of bonding through breastfeeding. It was something she thought she'd have to give up by adopting, and was still in awe that her body could do this with stimulation and supplements.

"Wow," Angie exclaims. "I did not know that you could do that!"

"Yes," I interject. "She is going to be the PT—preferred tit." Sallyann and I laugh knowingly, and Angie looks confused.

"You know how a little one seems to connect more with a particular parent?" I ask.

"Yes," she responds slowly.

"Well, we've joked that since Sallyann hasn't had an infant before, she will be our baby's PT. So we're aiming to do all we can to support that," I explain.

"I see. That's so cool. I am impressed by your diligence. How often do you pump?" Angie asks.

"Every two hours, and I have put him to my breast," Sallyann says. "He latches on great. It's such a natural form of comfort, you know, whether for feeding or not. It's good to get him used to it."

"He latched on when he was only about an hour old. He's a strong little guy," I say, kissing his head.

Again, Angie gestures to the bags. "Open! Open something."

"Here, Sallyann—you first." I hand her a bag, she sits on the edge of the bed near Angie, and pulls out a neatly wrapped item. Each bag has two or more packages. It is like a one-person mini baby shower.

Angie continues making a fuss over Sage, calling him Little Man and caressing his head.

"How adorable!" Sallyann holds up a little sleeper that is terry cloth, striped brown and white. There is a set of bibs in the box, too.

"He'll need something for the warmer days we might still get, and I love how terry washes easily and breathes." Angie is pleased, I can tell, with Sallyann's sincere appreciation of the gifts.

We take turns opening the sleepers, blankets, and small wrist rattles that have been so thoughtfully chosen and wrapped for us.

I love watching Sallyann as the center of attention. I would prefer she open everything, but she insists— no surprise to me—that we take turns. I love her glow. I love her laugh. She is so happy. She's always been a basically happy person since I've known her, not sappy-happy, but joy filled and deeply, richly contented. Even through the years of disappointment and failed attempts at pregnancy, she still had a joy in her soul that was unshakable. This is different, though. This is the dream-come-true, top-of-the-mountain, pure joy that happens only a few times in any lifetime. I can hardly believe we are here. It's been worth every fertility treatment, the classes, the home study, and whatever the final legal bill will be when this wraps up next month. It's worth the waiting, the hopefulness, and the disappointments to get here, to finally be with our little Sage man. Our family is complete. The real journey has begun.

TWO BOYS
Rebecca, 2001

"I have two boys and they have issues." Was I really saying this to someone I just met? Her eyes were so honest. It's as though I've seen her before, known her already, even though this is the first we've met.

"Really? Well, no one is perfect, I guess," she said, and blushed. I blushed, too.

I was not embarrassed; my face was certainly hot, though. She was stunningly beautiful and had a voice like a song—slightly gravelly, with a spontaneous laugh. I followed her from glass showcase to bookshelf, looking for a gift for a wedding, the reason I'd stopped into the store in the first place, Peace of Mind Emporium. She was a peaceful soul, or peace seeking, or perhaps both—I could sense it. I felt grounded and like I was floating at the same time.

"How old are these boys of yours?" she asked, lifting her eyes to meet mine over a case filled with small angel pins and bracelets.

"Five and seven . . . and a half. They both have birthdays in the spring, just a few weeks apart. I am lucky; they play really well together. Sometimes siblings are not so great together. They love to be outside, and that works for me. I love to garden, both veggies and flowers." I was rambling, I knew it, and wanted to stop. I was nervous, or excited, or something. She was smiling, and it was an incredible smile that compelled me to smile as well.

"Well, I think I will take that angel pin with the wings spread out. Her life has been tough, and I am not sure this marriage will help, so she may need an angel on her shoulder."

She took it out of the case and we moved toward the checkout area.

"Would you like it wrapped?" she asked, and I answered quickly, "Yes, please," mostly because I wanted more time with her. She carefully pulled a starry paper off the roll and wrapped, making a bow out of the curling ribbon.

"Thank you. It is beautiful."

We both blushed a bit again.

I had never believed in love at first sight. Maybe I hadn't been opening my eyes, or maybe I had never set sight on someone so lovable before.

That was only a few weeks before the Twin Towers fell. We didn't have real TV at our house, and I did all I could to be sure the boys did not watch the tragedy. Their world was already unstable: Both struggled in school. They traveled to their dad's every weekend, which included being with their very religious grandparents. Then they came back to our little double-wide trailer on a two-acre plot in rural Vermont. For months, I made all the ends meet by supplementing a full-time job in crisis work with being a cashier at the local general store while the boys were with their dad, from Saturday evening through Sunday morning. I was so tired when I picked them up on Sundays, I sometimes fell asleep while playing Robin Hood or pirates.

"The ship rocked me to sleep," I would say groggily.

I wanted more time with them. Over the three years since I'd divorced Peter, I had investigated how to create a way to spend every day without dropping them off with someone else. Seth awoke crying every night the first month I worked full-time. Finally, one night I made out the words between his sobs: "I miss you, Mommy." I cried with him. What a mess. I had created such a mess for the two little beings I cared so much for.

"How do you clean up such a complete mess?" I would shout at my extremely patient therapist, whom I had been seeing for five years.

"It will get better. You can create a life and the love that you want," Kat would calmly say, as if saying it would make it so.

She must not understand. She cannot see how inept I am, or how could she believe that?

If I ran my own daycare, it would be pretty much impossible to earn enough to feed us all.

Only after pages of applications and background checks and a house visit was I told that, yes, I'd been cleared to take in a disabled adult, which would pay over thirty thousand dollars per year. But I had to keep my full-time job. In addition, I had to have another viable means of support. *Seriously, then what was the point?* I wondered.

I attempted writing for money, but it was so difficult

with all the other spinning plates whirling on my fingertips. Writing to clear my head, that came easily, but not with any financial compensation. Words flowed into journals, years of pain that had been chained inside me. Locked in by my own hands and piles of shame. The place I was in was not something I was proud of at all. Coming from a Bible Belt family, divorce was not an option, and my parents didn't speak to me except to chastise for the first year after our split.

These boys, Sawyer and Seth, or Sugar and Cinnamon, as I dubbed them, rustling their hair—Sawyer's was pure blond and Seth's was very light brown—they were always on my mind.

Was it the right decision, leaving their father? Or was it a huge mistake that would leave scars running too deep to heal?

The boys' therapist, who they began to see a few weeks after Peter's breakdown, told me that children who are part of two households have two families to learn from. I tried to see any positives, but it did not erase the pain.

Somehow it was less lonely when there was no other adult in the house, rather than someone being there who I hoped to feel as a companion and having that need go unmet. As quiet as it was after the sun went down, and the only sounds were from the boys' rhythmic breathing and gentle snoring, it was lonelier by far to have been next to someone whose heart I could not connect with. To look at someone I thought I relied on and realize I was not seen at all. For me, this space was better—it was a peaceful place, though not perfect, not at all.

"Progress, not perfection," the instructor at the parenting class I was taking said. "Just progress. None of us are perfect, but we can make progress." This was hard to wrap myself around, when the past thirty years of Christianity had told me I must aspire to perfection, that anything less demanded punishment. It resonated with me, though. Each of us was unique. It made sense to work on building up these distinctive parts of the children rather than instilling them with the negativity that comes with constant punishment.

I went to the fridge, where a large sign read BREATHE, and instinctively wanted to scream about the spilled juice on the kitchen floor. Instinct that came from the rules and punishments of my own parents railing within my mind and heart, sown into my shame. I wanted something else for Sawyer and Seth, but it was not easy. It was painful when I let my scream land in their little ears, and I saw the look of shame and anger in their eyes. Remembering that look kept me glued to the sign, counting my breaths, in and out. It was painful to hold in, to not scream, to not hit them, and to not submit them or me to that pain. Where did I end and they begin? Where did I begin and my parents end?

Let the pain inflicted on each other end here. *Breathe.*

I went outside, smoked a cigarette, paced around the house. Breathed again. I walked down the driveway, up again, peeking in the windows. They were smiling and running Matchbox cars down the ramp Sawyer had made, sending the tiny cars flipping onto the carpet. I could hear Seth's laugh through the window and see Sawyer's eyes sparkling at the sound, as he did it again and again to entertain him.

Peace, laughter, joy. None of this is a given. It is work. It takes focus. But it was worth it when I saw their smiles.

I could not be with them every minute, but I could make every minute into as positive a memory as it could be. I was tired, it was getting dark. Maybe popcorn and a cartoon video were okay tonight. Maybe just feeling each other close was enough for the time being. Let the dishes soak, the juice remain on the floor, the Matchbox cars staying sticky too. We could clean together after we held each other close, and I knew that was more important than a clean floor. Life just isn't clean; it's so untidy.

I opened the door and their eyes landed on me, waiting for a sign. I smiled, they both smiled and giggled a bit, and I wondered aloud whether Matchbox cars would be fun in the bathtub. Both were game to see, and ran from kitchen to tub, piling them in. I started the water and added the bubbles.

DEBBIE'S INTERRUPTION
Sallyann, 2014

We haven't met the paternal grandmother or the biological father. What I know about them is hearsay and, even now, they don't seem to play a determining role.

I am far more concerned about Debbie, the maternal grandma, this woman who has not been invited by her daughter to be present during the birth, but who insisted on holding Sage during his first day on Earth, several times, even as her daughter was requesting not to see him. I am worried about a birth mother who is not ready to look at the baby she is eagerly giving away, but I check it off as her way of making it easier on herself, especially if he was conceived by rape, as she had disclosed to the hospital social worker and the lawyer. I am worried that Debbie is more focused on seeing and holding Sage than being with her daughter and supporting her through her vulnerability and loss.

I am especially concerned when the nurses return to us with reports of Debbie saying things to relatives in front of the nurses, such as, "I could bring him home and raise him as if he were *my* son. He'd *never* have to know that Delilah gave birth to him." That seems such a desperate statement, one that may speak to her desires but in no way seems to acknowledge what her daughter needs.

The nurses report that Debbie is reaching out to the paternal grandmother to get her involved, hoping her sway might make the biological father—or purported rapist—file to keep the baby. It's as if they are talking about someone else's child, not the one I have enveloped in my arms.

I could understand Debbie's desperation, her dream of keeping him rooted in his family of origin. But I could not stand to watch her manipulating so many people, especially her child, by overstepping Delilah's boundaries like that.

Rebecca makes frequent visits with Corey and Delilah while we are in the hospital together, always checking on the kids to see what support they need, to tell them what is available to them in the community. During one of these visits, Corey backs up what the nurses told us. It is true that someone had contacted the birth father's family, and now that boy's "crazy mother was posting shit all over Facebook about 'the little bitch who is keeping me from my grandson,'" Corey reported.

If it was proven to be rape, it didn't seem like these people had a wing or a prayer. Delilah's lawyer was already attempting to prosecute the birth father with rape charges. He'd lose all rights to the baby if the case was successful, and the grandmothers had no legal rights to this baby in the state of Vermont. If the birth mother wanted to give up the baby, it was her decision completely.

Should I have been more concerned by Corey and Delilah's anxiety when they reported to us on the afternoon after meeting Delilah's lawyer, alongside her mother, that Debbie "threw a fit" when she found out that "basically a grandmother has no right to her grandchild"? They told us that she got up, huffed away, and slammed the door behind her, even before they'd completed the visit with this professional, who we were paying for. This was a hotheaded woman.

She performed with niceties. But when it came down to a fight, she was a dog with a bone. She was not letting go. At all. "Delilah thinks this is gonna go down one way, but this is not gonna go the way she planned it"— another statement she'd made, this one directly to one of the nurses.

These nurses had seen it all. Most of this drama did not surprise them. Like us, they were impressed by Delilah's fortitude and her conviction that she was doing the right thing with her decision. We had to get signed permission for everything, including our ability to name Sage and whether to circumcise him, because Delilah held legal custody right now, even though she had signed over physical custody to us. Delilah signed everything without a second's hesitation.

The nurses were also impressed by our affection

with each other and Sage, by the fact that I am working on breastfeeding him and, in the interim, giving him organic formula, which he digests well. He is gaining weight. He is healthier than most infants they see on formula. They swear the organic formula, coupled with all the physical bonding we are giving him, mean so much for Sage's development. They seem surprised that we would commit ourselves to going the extra mile.

It does not feel like anything extra to me. He is my baby. He is my son. I know that, even if all I can give him from my nipple is, at the moment, a weak stream of colostrum; it is still so important for his development to suckle. I know it will provide him comfort and, as his mom, of course, I will comfort him. He is my love. He is our gift.

"Well, not to worry about Debbie," a nurse assures us. "There's a lot of hullabaloo coming from her, but the drama usually dies down once everyone is out of the hospital and back to their respective lives."

I smile, hoping she is right.

MEETING THE BOYS
Sallyann, 2002

People do not often ask, "Why do you want to have a baby?" But they think nothing of asking or judging couples who do not want babies. People in my world generally didn't ask when I got involved with Rebecca why I wanted to do that either, or why I would also be taking in her two boys. If the questions were there, if the concerns were there, they were rarely spoken aloud—except for my silvery-haired friend Sandy, who had adopted me as if I were one of her own. We'd weathered the death of her husband, Paul, whom I had grown to love dearly. We spent years looking out for each other as we checked in and shared creative hobbies and metaphysical interests.

Shortly after my involvement with Rebecca began, with all Sandy had learned about Rebecca's past, as well as her boys, Sandy played the voice of reason, expressing her concerns. "Maybe you'd want to wait before you move in with all of them." Sandy went on, "Are you actually sure you want to do this? I mean, you could get your own place and the two of you can still see each other and develop your relationship with the boys without jumping into the fire, so to speak. Do you feel that what you have with Rebecca is strong enough already?"

She folded her napkin in front of her and leaned forward. "I mean, let's just get real here," she said. "She comes with some real baggage. Her ex, for instance. He's got some heavy-duty problems, to say nothing about what that has done to their kids. And"—she paused and sat straight back in her chair—"clearly, her boys do have some issues. I mean it's not going to be an easy haul. The younger one—well, even you have thought he might be living at home until well into his thirties."

She stood up and walked to the kitchen and brought back a pot of tea to refill our mugs.

"Don't get me wrong. I think Rebecca is a lovely woman, and I know you cherish her, and rightfully so. And I'm glad she keeps you on a satin pillow, with your best interests at heart. But are you absolutely sure you want to take this all on? You're still quite young, and this is a huge commitment, and well, hard to say at this point how things can turn out for those boys, you know? They could go either way. They could grow up to be pretty difficult guys." I watched the fear fill her eyes as if she was envisioning a mean and angry future for me. "Or, of course, with the love and encouragement of two beautiful women like yourselves . . ." She did not complete the thought, and the brief silence allowed me to step in.

"I have given thought to all of this, Sandy," I reassured her. "I really have. This is why Rebecca and I are already ahead of the game and in counseling together, because we want this to be done as thoughtfully as possible with everyone's interests in mind. I really think what we have here so far can grow into something positive for us all. Do I know for sure? No. But Rebecca and I do stay in communication about our thoughts and feelings."

She looked at me with hesitation, not sure whether to believe I wasn't being all pie-in-the-sky lovey-dovey instead of two-feet-on-the-ground with my heart facing forward. Inside, I did feel as if I was defending my love for Rebecca, as well as our future. I was irritated by what felt more like a negative checklist, as opposed to applauding Rebecca's ability to point out the silver linings of life. But I also felt grateful Sandy was looking out for me, that she wanted to remind me I needn't give my power away this time, that there were still choices within the relationship I could make.

Rebecca's therapist, Kat, had been meeting with us for several months when we proposed a meeting date with the boys. I felt sick to my stomach; my nerves seemed to be combusting. I'd been in a relationship before that had involved kids. I didn't want to attach to these guys only to lose them, as I had with those children. But would these boys even accept me? How would getting to know them change my relationship with Rebecca? Kat, Rebecca, and I worked out a low-key plan, where I would get to see them in person but we wouldn't be confessing our undying love to them. I knew Rebecca was cautious, guarded around her boys with her intimate relationships, not wanting to involve them in anything else that would hurt them, and I respected that as much as I respected that she was up front in telling me she had two boys the first day I met her. She warned me several times that her boys had issues, and I knew how she'd interrupted her workday to go to the elementary school they were in at the time to change the clothes of the six-year-old who kept having accidents. I knew her eight-year-old used to throw tantrums after her divorce, that he could be very difficult, and a bit like his dad. I'd seen their photos. They were darling little towheads with wide-eyed expressions and soft blue eyes.

Because I'd been to their home, though they were not there at the time, I'd seen their toys, their dress-up costumes, their automobile fabric curtains she'd made them, and their bunk beds. I'd smelled the lingering odor of a urine-soaked mattress that had been laboriously cleaned but still held its mark. I'd seen the trail of Legos on the floor, and I'd even felt the boys' leftover energies—raw, rambunctious, somewhat erratic. Without meeting them, I could sense a hauntedness they brought back from visits to their dad's family, a wariness that was inherent to their trauma.

We had agreed to meet up at the Pizza Hut in town to have dinner with the boys and then, if all went well, I would join them afterward at the school's Scholastic book tour. I knew they loved books, which at least gave us some shared ground. I knew very little about small boys, despite being the eldest cousin of so many boys, despite playing with them when they were little tykes. I felt intimidated, as if I'd have nothing much in common with them. They sounded like unique little buggers and, as much as I loved little kids and had an affinity for the gifted, I still wasn't sure I could hold my own. I felt nearly as young as them, in some ways.

Sawyer had these convincing icy-blue eyes that sparkled with curiosity and assuredness. He launched into a detailed description of his favorite book series, the Animorphs. I could hardly take my eyes off him. He was bright and extremely articulate. He spoke didactically, like a little professor engrossed in his topic. His newfound passion for books—Rebecca told me he had struggled with reading until recently—was contagious to me; it was a bond we could easily cement.

Her younger son, Seth, sat across from us, quietly eating his pizza, laughing when his brother laughed, his head mostly down, intent on the food he was chewing. I'd actually seen Seth once before, at a housewarming party held after Rebecca moved into the home we would eventually share. She'd suspected he was autistic, like her sister's son, though differently affected. Seth was adorable, with an effervescent grin and soft, emanating light-blue eyes that were faraway, seemingly gazing upon another planet. He had walked amongst the crowd of adults as if they were ghosts surrounding him. Because I knew it was important to get to know him, I'd followed him into his room, where he was repeatedly smacking down a Beanie Baby, making whooshing and bombing noises as he did. He did not say much to me, and when he did start to speak he would begin his sentence again and again, each time adding an additional word. It was painstaking and exhausting. He was a bundle of leaping, flying energy, but it was obvious he was in his own world and I was not really there with him, even if he answered a question of mine. I felt lonely for us both.

At Pizza Hut, I was gladdened to see that Seth looked up toward his mom and pointed things out to her in a gentle, high-pitched voice. It was also evident he adored his older brother, whose words were the only ones he hung on to.

I listened to and observed them, and watched Rebecca with them, ever vigilant, looking for behaviors that might indicate her sons were as sociopathic as her older brother sounded, whether they were as messed up as she sometimes made it sound like they were. And I was aware of the family unit they all were. They functioned together like one organism, better than I'd seen a lot of kids with their moms.

I'd better like them, I thought, because I knew it was a deal breaker for our relationship if I did not. Rebecca had once said that she couldn't imagine being in a relationship with someone who didn't love her kids as much as she loved them. Her words seemed a tall order to me. Could I aspire to that? Could anyone? She talked about her boys a lot. She loved sharing stories about playing Maid Marian to their Robin Hood, about their inventiveness and their logic. At night when we spoke on the phone, I heard their voices in the background. She would interrupt our conversation to cut them apples when they requested. I'd hear her soft voice soothingly sending them off toward bed. These boys were her world.

Rebecca's boys were not just her reflection but people she saw as future adults, who she respected and admired, even when they drove her crazy.

It was watching her with her boys that made me feel I could learn from her, and maybe parenting with her could be safer than it had been in my previous relationship. And if somebody ever asked me why I wanted a baby, I would eventually be able to say it was because I really enjoyed being a parent with Rebecca, even though it took a while to get to the point where it felt more rewarding than not. We could bear the burden together, against the odds and despite them.

THE BABYSITTER'S HERE
Sallyann, 2014

I pick up my cell phone. There is a message from our lawyer: "Hey, ladies. This is Irene Haines calling. Can you give me a call back?"

I missed the call because I'd been curled up on the couch, rocking Sage in my arms. From the moment we arrived home nearly a week ago, our home has been a revolving door of friends and relatives, starting with our dear friend Sarah who greeted us as we pulled in and helped us remove him from the conundrum that was the infant car seat.

My uncle Steve had just left. He stopped over to meet our little guy and, in his usual behavior, greeted us with an exclamatory waving of hands and full-body gestures as he told us excitedly about his latest gig as the football game announcer for the college where I worked. When I finally released Sage into his arms, he held him awkwardly at first; it did not feel as natural to him as a football or basketball, but he was doing his best. There was a tender glint in his eyes as he looked down and spoke softly to our little guy. I helped arrange Sage in his arms until I could see body memory take over. Yes. He'd had a baby boy once. Uncle Steve's son was twenty-five now. I remembered the first time I'd met my cousin, Cade, that summer before we first moved to Vermont. I was fourteen and he was a bouncy six-month-old, all eyelashes and cheeks and baby blue eyes that turned greener as he aged.

As Steve fussed over Sage, I watched the hopefulness in Steve's soft blue eyes. I could imagine our uncle trying to teach him how to block a pass or—deep breath in—run the football. I could see Steve raising his arms—"Touchdown!"—and Sage responding, as a toddler, his arms raised to the sky. These sports were not necessarily the scenarios I pictured for our little man. With his long, curling fingers, I imagined a pianist or a string musician. That was just my bias, of course.

I know he will have so much to ask from life and his future, and I am grateful he'll get to experience the people I love. I picture our friends Kim and Matt, who are coming to see him that afternoon with their ten-year-old twins, and later, our dear friend Roxie. Our house has had quiet times since his arrival, moments with just the three of us which we soak up, like little sponges of love. But it is also a fount of activity, a revolving door of friends and family, of excited, exuberant faces that can barely wait to get their arms around Sage, who hug us in celebration—wholehearted hugs. Joy bursts over the seams of the windows and doorways. It is better than any holiday. We have the best gift in town, the one we can all share.

I imagine Sage learning funky crafts and vegetarian dishes from Kim, great Lego ideas and engineering concepts from Matt. I imagine that little Henry and Ella might eventually become trusted sitters for him. I think back to holding them as infants, feeling shy and awkward with them in my arms, as my uncle had just seemed. I think of Roxie teaching him to be politically active, to build a revolution, to dance his heart out to tribal rhythms.

But who knows what he will learn from these people? Ultimately, his lessons are his own, and the important thing is that he will be safe and he will be cherished. Isn't that what any reasonable person wants for their baby? Wouldn't it be grand if we could all come into the world welcomed by loving arms, kept emotionally, mentally, and physically safe? If all needs could be met?

My heart ricochets off the walls of my throat. Why is our lawyer calling on a Sunday afternoon? *Has the court date for the termination of parental rights been changed again?* I quietly hope. It was moved from Friday to Monday after Corey and Delilah had transportation issues and couldn't make it on the original date. Maybe there needs to be another adjustment. Or perhaps there is an update on the birth father. We know from Delilah's lawyer that he was urged by his mother to file for paternity testing. Again, that isn't something that needs to be addressed on Sunday. But there is urgency in her voice.

I take a deep breath in and dial the number she left for me.

"I'm so sorry."

When your lawyer greets you with this language, you know you're facing a stream of words you do not want to ever hear her utter.

"Jenifer, Delilah's lawyer, contacted me. Delilah wants the baby back. Maybe you could call her. She might be having postpartum feelings, you know?"

A shockwave. A tornado. A blast.

I am sitting, feeling his warm body against my heart, watching as he tucks himself toward me.

But all around me, all around us, the walls are disintegrating.

Surely I am not hearing her correctly.

Surely this can be changed.

"I don't have her phone number." I hear myself utter sounds that I know are comprehensible, but they make no sense to me.

Rebecca is at my side, her eyes dilating as she hears my voice. I can see pain work its way into her features.

"Oh," Irene said, "I must have misunderstood. I thought you'd known each other and were in communication before the baby was born."

"Yes," I breathe. "We were in communication via our friend Cheryl, but only for a week. We never exchanged phone numbers with Delilah. We had tried to maintain appropriate boundaries throughout all our interactions, to give her a respectful space and give us privacy. It made sense for all of us to have some boundaries."

"Okay. Well, you will need to call Jenifer and see if Delilah gives you permission to call her directly. Jenifer can then give you her number."

I could not fashion a coherent thought. My brain was a box of jumbled crayons.

Jenifer who? I thought. *Delilah who?*

That foolish wench, Delilah, you mean? That false

giver?

Some giveth, some taketh away.

She was doing both to us.

I follow Irene's order and obtain Delilah's phone number from Jenifer.

"I don't know if I can do it," I tell Rebecca. "I don't know if I can call her."

Neither of us wants to touch the phone; it has become the hot potato between us.

I can see Rebecca's gears going, doing what she always does, trying to fix this.

"Maybe she just needs to see him," she echoes Irene. "Maybe she's having postpartum emotions. She might just want to know he's okay." I nod. I want her to be right. I also know she is trying desperately to convince us both.

I take another deep breath in, and dial.

Corey answers.

At the sound of my voice, he gives a casual, "Oh, hi," as if I'd called five minutes before, or was calling to talk about the weather, check in on his day.

"Hi, Corey. Is Delilah available?"

"Sure." Maybe he is as anxious as I am, but there is no "Let me get her," no "How are you guys?" Better yet, "How's the baby?" He is such a kid himself.

"Delilah, I received a call from our lawyer. She says you want the baby back. What happened? What has made you change your mind?"

Inside I am crying out: *Whhhhyyyyyyyyyyyyyyyyyy?*

Her response comes out stilted, as if she is a robot.

"I just want to raise my son."

Ouch.

It is the first time I hear her refer to him as *her son*. Before, he was a distant, almost inanimate object, or "the baby."

"But why? Why now? What has changed?" I can hear the pleading in my voice.

Again, she repeats the script as if reading it from a teleprompter.

"I just want to raise my son."

My whole body shakes. How dare she call him that *now*. She wanted no part in this nine days ago. She has not held him, fed him, bathed him, sung to him, kissed his fuzzy head, changed him, breastfed him. She wanted us to make all the decisions. Whenever the nurses had asked, she'd sent them to us with paperwork: Would he be circumcised? Would he be okay to receive his vaccinations?

She told her instructor at school that she would leave him at the hospital after the birth; she had no intention of raising a child. She had not once—and we'd checked again and again—not once indicated that she wanted to keep him.

And we want him with all our hearts.

I can't help but wonder if her mother is standing over her as she takes this call because the message we've gotten from her mother is far different.

I hear myself speak. "When do you want him?"

At some point, I hear her respond that she wants him tomorrow.

Tomorrow? If you want him so badly, why aren't you

asking for him *now*?

Tomorrow? So, you're going to give us twenty-four hours to say goodbye, then?

"But you don't have anything, do you?" I am desperately clutching onto any reason why she can't take him. "Do you have diapers, stroller, clothes, formula?" I list, mentally checklisting everything we'd saved up for, purchased, collected from others. I want to ask, "Do you really love him? Why are you doing this to him?"

But all I can focus on are the items to meet his needs.

Again comes her only refrain: "I want to raise my son."

I am blubbering now and cannot talk. Rebecca is watching me intently through this, intermittently biting the inside of her cheek.

I hand her the phone. I am crying too hard to continue. It is all I can do not to lunge at the phone, as if it were Delilah in person.

Apparently, she is as resolute now at saying nothing as she had been about handing him over to us.

Oh, wait. She isn't handing him over.

She is taking him back.

Rebecca reiterates the same questions I asked, receives the same response.

Somehow, we make an arrangement with the help of our lawyer and hers, and decide we can meet at a neutral spot—our lawyer's office—the next day at noon. There, we would handle the exchange.

The exchange. What are we doing? A drug deal? Parental custody visits? It's all so surreal.

I look at the time.

Our friends are coming soon. But how can we see them now? How can we introduce them to our boy, our boy who is leaving our arms forever in just twenty-four hours? Rebecca calls Kim and explains what is happening. She tries to talk Kim and Matt out of coming, but they are already out the door. They still want to see us, they say. They won't stay, but they want to bring us some food they've made.

Hours later, after they've left, before our next friend comes to visit, I decide to call my parents. Of the many people we would now have to share this news with, my parents' voices are two of the most difficult for me to hear.

I can still see their doting eyes in my mind's eye, the way they held our Sage, their presumed grandbaby. I was stunned by their attachment, their affection, our group adoration of this sweet little guy.

My father's words are in the background, as the news breaks like egg and oozes into the air around us. I hear the notes of contempt, a familiar wash of his pain and anger, mixed and rushing: "So now you're basically a glorified babysitter?"

If Delilah's words stabbed me in the chest, his words kick me in the gut and take the wind right out of me.

Babysitter?

I am his mom.

I will never be his babysitter.

Yet, there it is, the truth to his statement. Essentially, we are watching *her* baby now, while she gathers the items she needs to care for him.

I look at Sage in Rebecca's arms, all squished up against her, all warm and snuggly. I can smell his forehead from here—his scent embedded in my mind and in my heart.

I wonder if Delilah is being pushed into this, wonder if there is anything we can do to change her mind. Then I hear Rebecca raising her own doubts, giving voice to my thoughts about all the things we could have, should have done differently since we'd left the hospital.

This is turning into an abrupt climax. Gone are all the bells and gongs of celebration that we experienced for the past week.

I ask my parents if they want to see him once more, want to say goodbye. They do not. They act as if they are giving us the benefit of being alone with him to say our farewells. But they've come to see him nearly every day since his birth. Their willing absence now reverberates around us.

SHELTER KISS
Rebecca, 2003

It was a warm spring day, and climbing out of bed to come to work was getting easier with more sunlight. The smokers were all gathered on the porch. I liked to stand and chat with them, even though I stopped smoking two years ago. I sometimes held a pen or other object, just for the sense of inclusion. Funny how that got ingrained even in just three years as a smoker. Jokingly, I asked Kimberly for a cigarette. She knew Sallyann would not support my nicotine fetish.

"*No*, I will not. What would Sallyann say?"

"Just kidding." I laughed.

She knew it; I just loved to get a reaction.

Leslie came out onto the porch. She never hung out with us here, so I knew something was up. "I need to talk with you, Rebecca," she said firmly.

Leslie didn't ask to see me often. Not alone, outside of a regular staff meeting. It made me a little nervous. I followed her to the director's office in the next building, a small, narrow room that used to be a porch. It was piled high with extra pillows for women arriving with nothing in the middle of the night. They showed up missing a shoe, their wallet, or a nightgown. A large trunk contained new pajamas, underwear, and an assortment of bras donated by a women's organization in town.

We sat across from each other, she in her desk chair and I in a soft, overstuffed seat.

"I wanted you to understand that you can't be kissing Sallyann on shelter property."

"Excuse me?" I said, startled. I was not sure I was hearing her right—I couldn't be. What the hell did she mean? It was none of her damn business.

"If you are going to be director, you need to know that this town is not ready for a lesbian director. It is too conservative. It just won't fly. You will lose funding." Leslie was firm.

What was she saying? Was she out of her mind? Really, was she serious? I think she was. But who would stop funding us?

"I got a phone call yesterday from our neighbor, Diane. She asked me if I knew you were a lesbian. I told her it was none of my business, or hers. So I want you to know I headed that off, but you can't be so public." She was looking down at papers on her desk.

"I can't be public?" My voice rang with disbelief. Leslie looked exasperated. I met the firm tone of her voice. "Leslie, you have kissed Barney in and outside the shelter; why would this be any different?

She sighed like a mother whose child won't clean her room. "But it is different. Very different. This is a very conservative town." She raised her voice a notch. "You need to understand this if you want to be director."

"Are you saying you don't think I should be director if I am a lesbian?" I said, appalled.

"No, no not at all. That isn't what I mean." She became

more emphatic, but I was sure this was exactly what she did mean.

"So, you are saying I just need to hide the fact that I am a lesbian?" I said directly.

"Yes, exactly. You can't be so public about it. It is in the best interest of the shelter." She smiled, pleased that I was getting it.

Really? *Really?*

"Then perhaps it is in the best interest of the shelter if I am not the director." I began to stand.

"No, no, that isn't necessary." Now Leslie was shocked.

"Yes, Leslie, it is." I was firmer than I knew I could be. Our eyes met. "I am who I am. I had to hide for years. I was ashamed of who I am for years. I won't do that. I won't do that now," I stated with no hesitation.

There was silence between us. The room seemed darker than ten minutes ago. I heard muffled street noise, a woman singing to her infant on the other side of the wall, inside the shelter's living room. My mind was swirling.

What would I do? What other job could I find? Will we need to move?

"I kiss her anywhere anyone else would kiss their lover, the one they are married to, or in a relationship with. I kiss her on dates, on our back porch . . ."

"*On your porch?*" she interrupted, her eyes growing wide. Then she took a breath. "You shouldn't do that," Leslie added emphatically.

"Why? Why, Leslie, why shouldn't I?" I was aghast.

"Your boys . . . think of them. You should think of them and what they will have to go through in school if their classmates know you are a lesbian," she stated.

"Leslie, what will my boys have to go through if they have a mother who isn't proud of who she is? How will they be proud of who they are if they think I am ashamed of who I am? That makes no sense at all to me. They will learn to stand up for who they are and what they believe, if they see it. Not if they see me acting differently in private and in public." I was certain of my stance.

Six years of Leslie's stories came to me in a flood: Telling her teen children that the dryer was broken so they wouldn't waste electricity by drying a single pair of jeans; putting her adopted daughter, who'd stolen from her, out on the porch, in a blizzard, and her husband, Barney, taking her back inside; advising me that if the insurance on the trampoline was too expensive at our new house, perhaps I could "lose" parts of it in the move.

No, I had lived enough lies. It wasn't part of who I was anymore. Adding to my shame, I'd had to shelter my brother and protect my minister ex-husband from my shame—and this was too important to be drowned in my shame. Not when I was starting a relationship that was so very important to me. I loved Sallyann. I loved Sallyann more than anyone on this planet. It had been only two years; people will think I am crazy, I was sure.

I wanted this to work. I wanted it to work because Sallyann was amazing. I wanted to shout to the whole neighborhood that she was my beloved and I was so thrilled. She met me halfway. She carried half the load. She was a real partner. She stayed home with Sawyer or Seth if they were sick. She showed up! I didn't want dark shades pulled over this bright, shining love. Who would? Heterosexuals didn't have to. They could hold hands and kiss each other in public, and we'd all smile. We weren't disrobing or anything. My god, it wasn't even a deep kiss. It was just a quick kiss—okay, maybe a brief kiss on the lips, but Christ. Really?

Our eyes were locked, Leslie's and mine. It felt as if we had been in this silence for hours, not minutes.

I broke the silence.

"If you want to reconsider my position as assistant director and consider hiring someone else to replace you, that is fine. Not kissing my beloved wherever we are, that is not fine."

I turned to the door. I walked out. I closed the door carefully behind me, even though I would have so loved to slam it. I was still shocked. So shocked, I was not sure what had really just happened.

LAST DAY
Sallyann, 2014

If you've read about numerology, you know that numbers are given spiritual and symbolic significance. Like sacred geometry, there are patterns and relationships between numbers, as well as inherent codes. One is very different from two, we all know, and it's certainly different from three, or five, or a thousand—whether counting money or counting stars. In numerology, the number nine signifies the end of a cycle. This makes sense in the logic of numbers, since, after nine we move on from single digits to double digits. The form changes shape.

But who cares about numerology when time has given way to seconds? Each second a seed, where Sage rocks in our arms, wriggles in his moose-covered onesie, breathes against our chests, and murmurs soft sounds— sounds he will make for only a short time more before they become larger, louder, eventually deeper. On day nine we huddle close together, trying to beat the clock. On day nine, I watch the Earth speed around the sun, the axis change, the continents drift. I share him—but only with my beloved now. There is no one else here tonight. Only the three of us. And soon, it is just the two of us, as I rock in the recliner, holding him to my heart.

I stay up all night holding him, knowing it will be the last time we have together, those last moments that I can live in the fantasy of being his mom.

How have fantasy and reality blurred so much in a matter of weeks? At one point he was our dream, and then he became real. But soon he will be just a dream again. A memory.

I am determined to stay awake with him; actually, I can't even think about the concept of sleep. He is such an amazing gift to us all. And holding him, we already know how vast and irreplaceable every second is. We've sent two boys off already, and we'd watched them take on the forms of young men. We've seen the seasons pass and known the loss of other loved ones. We've celebrated holidays, weddings, other babies born, their graduations and weddings. The moment's magnitude falls upon us like a ton of bricks. After all, how do you part with your beloved? Nine days seems so short a span for an emerging love.

As I rock him, I lift him to my nose so I can take in his fresh baby scent, so buttery rich and faintly peach. I remind myself that when all is said and done, life is a treasure trove of moments, of memories, a blur of images that engage our senses; we attach and reengage, our neurons firing and misfiring.

It isn't the first time I've misfired on a fantasy, and, as

long as I'm alive, I know it won't be the last. My mind engages a false hope born of imagination, desire, and shock—that we really won't have to give him up, that just as surely as she'd changed her mind, she'll change it back again.

I want that dream so badly, I keep reimagining it, keep refocusing with a laser depth that is beyond obsessive. It is the switch that turns my mind on. Any thought to the contrary simply turns it off. And then—aha! A moment passes and it returns, and I rejoice internally each time because I am seeing him returned to my arms, to our arms, our very expectant arms.

But there is that incessant clock, meting out our seconds together. It is so intrusive. I keep trying to bid it farewell, but it just won't go away. You get only so many chances. You have only so much time with anyone. I think about how time is always stealing from us: youth, memories, people loved, and finally, life. Now it has returned to claim our baby and whisk our dreams away.

I begin telling him what I want him to know.

It's my job, after all, isn't it? I am still the parent, the guide. And there's so much ahead of him that I will never see. And I want to prepare him, and I want to protect him. And I am helpless to do either.

Ultimately, that is the truth, whether he is with me every day for the rest of his life or gone from me in the next breath.

I try to tell him, gently and quietly so his heart and his ears take it in: You will learn, if you are to grow.

You are sure to encounter struggle and hardship. You are certain to experience grief. You will be experiencing it early in your life, so you are already learning these lessons so young. And I'm sorry for that. But just know that I am infusing you with our love, with our hope, with our strength, so that in your every heartbeat and your every step on earth you know I am with you. And that we have loved you. That attention and affection will not ever go away.

Later, our friend Trish, a parent of three adopted children, will remind us how crucial the early developmental stages of life are and how meaningful to his life was all the love and attention that were showered on him. She'll say, "He was lucky to have experienced the degree of attention to his every need, which you gave him. There are so many people, so many babies, who never experience that." And we'll nod in agreement, because what else could we do? We also knew the science, the research about the growing mind, about the development of humanity. Oh, I thought, we all have such a long way to go if we are really going to grow.

What growth will he know? We will not see it, not even from afar. We just have to trust in his preciousness.

My foot presses the floor as I push from the rocking chair, push us further and further into the universe, where his sweet heart presses against mine . . . and all the love, all these moments I have carried deep in my heart . . . I try to give them to him. I surround him with them. And the seconds pass us by . . .

Every ounce of time weighs us down, in direct proportion to the distance from our destination and the loosening of the seconds. I watch his fingers loosen and grip, in a rhythm that matches that damned march forward.

Here I am, standing in formation, back straight, head upheld. Left, left, left, right, left. I march around with him like I am carrying a feather that will soon be lifted with the wind.

I begin to detach, to float away from myself. As I lay him down on the changing table. As I lift him up and kiss his little forehead. As I wrap him in his receiving blanket and swaddle him against me.

I feel the delicate weight of him warming my chest. But I am also watching myself rocking him. Listening to myself humming to him. How could anyone take this moment away? The world is full of such tender pictures as this—divine images of Mary holding Jesus, sacred photos of a babe in her mother's arms. I am immersed in the painting, and I am objectively viewing it. Meanwhile, every motion I make moves us forward in time, pushes us closer to noon—that other witching hour, that twelve o'clock when the ball will drop. I grow heavier, super sloth, moving as if both in fast-forward and rewind.

Rebecca and I give him the last bath together. And again, I keep telling myself: *No, this isn't the last time. Not really. Because he will return to us. Because that's how it's supposed to be.* We ease the lavender bodywash from our trip to Seattle onto our warmed hands, and we caress his skin as I look into his wide eyes, looking upward. I hope he feels surrounded by our love. That's all I could ever hope with anyone, but even I know that I was often immune to feeling the love of others, especially those who loved me the most. Who was to say it was sinking in to his every pore? Who was to say it wasn't?

We'd agreed to arrive with him at noon at a neutral spot, our lawyer's office.

I inch into the backseat with him, just as I have every time we have driven somewhere together. While Rebecca is in the driver's seat, I pay close attention to his every breath and murmur, squished up tightly in the car seat. And I am with him, with Rebecca, and not with either of them. I am drifting with the *thump-thump* of the car's tires, with the changing shape of the sky and its fiendish autumn glow. We are taking our time. The lawyer texted to let us know we should take our time, because Delilah has arrived with her mom, who is in a state.

Oh, really? I think. What audacity. *She* is in a state? What in the world did that mean? I picture her carrying on, screaming at lawyers whom she blamed for putting her family through this ordeal, kicking over trash cans, and cursing at people because she felt robbed of her grandbaby. If anybody should be in a state, shouldn't it be us? We are unearthly quiet, our breath barely audible, an eerie silence before a tornado.

So, I am just supposed to turn this peaceful baby over to some woman whose biology trumped any link I have to him? This woman who is, from the sound of it, having the temper tantrum of a two-year-old while our lawyer endeavors to calm her, to prevent a scene, and to protect us at the same time. Every physical urge in my body is telling me to fight back, to protect him from this. I am feeling the sheer terror of not knowing how I am going to let him go and what I am letting him go to. I have no power. Just as with this riotous grandma, there is not one iota of legal rights on my side.

Rebecca and I half-joked about running off to Canada with him, going into hiding, starting our lives over. We knew the outcome would mire us forever. We could never do that to Sawyer and Seth, to our friends and family. The legal consequences would be too great for us anyway. But what will be the consequences of releasing him to this birth family? How is that any less cruel of us, when we suspect that this is not entirely what his birth mother wants, when we know there is a potential rapist in the picture, and the other parties we'd met . . . do they have his best interests at heart? How can we deny him the abundance of love our family has and would provide? Can they give him the love, the safety, the reassurance of a good life that we knew we can give him? What are the guarantees of that? Are there any?

Finally, I see Irene exit from the front door of her office and move briskly toward our car. She is all apologies, sympathetic for what we are all about to do. By then, I had unhooked him from his car seat and am holding him against me, sustaining every moment I can with our little bundle, conscious of every breath between us, desperate to elongate what we have together. I can feel Rebecca's presence beside me, along with pressing pain in the bones of our chests, as if we are one body. Irene reaches into the car to take him from me and I begin to cry, a silent, oozing cry that emerges from another world. I can barely loosen my grip on him. I can hardly hand him over. But I watch myself doing it, watch from afar as she tucks him carefully into her arms. I watch as Rebecca hands over a bag of items for him, essentials we know he'll need.

My baby.

Our baby.

Our dreams.

Our hopes.

Our memories.

Our little guy.

He is going.

He is going—

He is gone.
And with him goes all the air around us.
And in its place—a vacuum emerges.

PART FOUR

Lose what I lose to keep what I can keep

MOVING DAY
Rebecca, 2015

Downsizing from 1,400 square feet to 192 is tricky. What do you bring, what do you store, and what is given away? Sallyann and I have lived in our Vermont home for fourteen years, and now it is a series of piles made with purpose, boxes filled with the most precious items that are being placed in the attic of the garage. Items we deem essential will be sent to Florida to become part of the new home we chose last week: a house on wheels, an eight-by-twenty-four-foot RV, though not for recreation in this instance. It is our new life. Sometimes life is so devastating that running away from home is the best option. So we are running.

It is bittersweet. I am helping our twenty-one-year-old son, Sawyer, who recently graduated from college, pack up his bedroom's accumulation of the past fourteen years. Sawyer is six foot, three inches and lanky, a perfect computer-geek stereotype. He looks at objects I hold up as if they are from another planet.

"Keep, store, or toss?" I ask for the hundredth time.

"Is that *mine*?" He looks so overwhelmed, a part of me wishes we weren't attempting to do all this in three weeks. Another part of me is glad to get it done, and done quickly. As if, like a child, I believe it will be less painful if I rip off the Band-Aid fast.

Sawyer has been a saint. With only the company of two cats, he stayed here alone for five weeks while Sallyann and I tried to get our bearings in faraway Florida. He job searched on his computer in this big, empty space, where he was used to the sounds of music, laughter, and all four of us. Meant to be all five of us. Had hoped to be five.

Sawyer had been so adorable holding his little brother of six days, Sage. I had no idea he was attached to babies, fascinated with their tininess, like me and Sallyann.

"Is he ours?" He asked the question quietly, Sage asleep in his arms.

"He *will* be ours," I emphasized, hoping the adoration Sawyer poured onto this little brother, twenty-one years younger, would stick with him. "Just in time for Thanksgiving. I can't imagine anything I could possibly be more thankful for," I said, looking at the small calendar hanging on the fridge. "Three happy, healthy boys. Is there anything better?"

I rubbed Sawyer's dirty-blond hair and joined him on the couch. Sage made little smacking noises. Sawyer and I looked at each other and giggled.

"He makes the cutest sounds," Sawyer exclaimed.

"I didn't know you liked babies so much," I said, stroking Sage's soft little finger, curled delicately around Sawyer's larger pointer finger.

"Oh yeah, it's cool when there is a new Hampden kid," he'd said, referring to his best friend's nieces and nephews who were born within the past few years to the crew of eight siblings.

"Right, I usually don't see you there, since you've driven yourself for the past five years," I added, and thought of the large Hampden family with their acres of farmland that included part of a mountain.

"Always something newborn on the farm." He grinned. "Calves, kittens, puppies, babies. Hey"—he paused—"when will he be old enough for me to read to him?"

"Now." I smiled.

"Seriously?" His expression was priceless, as if he'd just won a prize.

"Yes. I read to you while you were still in my tummy." I rubbed my stomach as if he were still in there.

"I have *Redwall* in my bag. Can I read him *Redwall*, or is that not appropriate yet?" He grinned. "It's my favorite."

"Of course you can read him *Redwall*. Let me grab it for you." I headed to the entry hall and took his backpack off the pegboard with SAWYER across it. I pictured another pegboard attached, about two feet off the floor, with SAGE in clear black lettering to match his big brothers' individualized coatracks. My mouth couldn't help but smile at the thought. I could see the boys when they were four and six years old, when they first got the little pegs to hang their belongings on at the door. These same pegs were much lower then, to match their reach. So, over the years, they were raised. We were shocked how quickly the coats started touching the floor, and up they would go again.

I put the pack next to Sawyer, and he directed me to the pocket with his well-loved book. No dog-ears, I thought. Sawyer always used a bookmark so as not to damage the pages. We all love reading, so bookmarks are abundant in this house.

"Here we go." I placed the book strategically in his hands so Sage was disturbed as little as possible.

"Okay, Sage, you don't have to love it, but you probably will." He opened and read the title and author before diving in to chapter one.

"He will be ours by Thanksgiving," I had assured him—I had lied.

Then I had left him all alone to housesit the space that Sallyann and I now couldn't bear to be in without feeling like the very soul of the home had been sucked out.

Sawyer held down the fort for us in the place we called home from the time he was in third grade and his brother Seth was in first.

I recalled so many wonderful Christmases with Sawyer awake first—well, sometimes Sallyann—eyes bright at the gifts surrounding the tree. Sallyann loved playing elf and handing out stockings first, full of sweet treats and Lego men, always a little Beanie Baby peeking over the edge. The stockings, from the Vermont Country Store, were each embroidered with a different holiday scene, stitched at the top with *Sawyer*, *Seth*, *Mom*, and *Sallyann*.

"I can look for work from anywhere," he'd said confidently. As a recent graduate from Rochester Institute of Technology, trying to find appropriate work and stay in Vermont was harder than he had imagined. He could feel our loss. The day after Sage left us, Sawyer helped move out all the Sage effects, while Sallyann disappeared into the bedroom.

We were too grief-stricken to think of how Sawyer might feel.

He felt our sobs; he knew how much I had cried the day before he left for college, and that was a happy occasion. But it *was* a huge change, a loss of the boy and the entrance of the man. Before he'd departed, I cooked his favorite breakfast, lunch, and dinner, and must've hugged him a hundred times, burying my face in his shoulder . . . Well, okay, closer to his ribs, since he is a foot above my five foot two.

Sawyer knew there was no time of day or night that was off-limits to his call, those times in high school and at college that he called on Mom for reassurance. "Am I good enough?" As he applied to colleges.

Sometimes for information: "How do you wash a tie?"

Or just to sort out priorities when the semester was mounting on him and he forgot to sleep, eat, or drink enough water.

Now he supported us, calling every few days to report on the cats, while we contemplated what would come next. "Boo-boo is poking me awake to feed her— right in the face, the little twerp. Pepper's mostly still hiding, but she actually sat by my foot yesterday."

We had lost Sawyer once, when we took a family-moon to Hawaii after our civil union in 2006. Poor

Sawyer caught a nasty cold on the first leg of the flight and felt miserable the first couple of days, but he was a good sport about it, especially once he and Seth hit the beach, only a block from the hotel.

With perfect waves on soft sand and almost bathwater temperatures, they rode their new Boogie Boards until we practically dragged them in, often taking water to them to be sure they stayed hydrated. Our treasured friend Kimberly, with whom I worked at the time, joined us on the trip to watch the boys for us in the evenings so Sallyann and I could enjoy dinner cruises and walk along Waikiki Beach.

The second day on the beach, we put our towels and supplies down while the boys went straight toward the water, along with hundreds of other tourists who were enjoying the perfect day. Sallyann, Kimberly, and I relaxed in the sun, munched on snacks, laughed together.

After an hour, the tide shifted a bit and we moved our setup about 100 feet to avoid the incoming waves and crowds. With the boys going in and out with the waves, their blond heads up and down all day, in and out of sight, the three of us continued our chatting, reading, and company for several hours. Finally, Seth came in for a snack, and we looked for Sawyer to see what he might want to eat. Then, we looked more. The waves were full of Boogie Boards, swimmers, bobbing heads, and people of all ages, but Sawyer was nowhere to be seen.

Stay calm, I told myself while fear mounted inside my entire being, heart, and soul.

Kimberly headed out to the water. I headed to the

lifeguard stand. Sallyann went up the beach further. We all directed Seth to stay on the towels. Every minute the panic inside rose. The lifeguards let me use their binoculars, but I did not see Sawyer's blond head among the swarms of people in the waves.

"Relax," a lifeguard assured us. "We keep a tight watch and haven't seen anyone distressed. I am sure he is fine."

Of course the lifeguard was sure; this wasn't *his* child.

It wasn't a part of *his* heart running around out there in the waves.

Nearly an hour passed and still no sign of Sawyer. Sallyann went to our hotel room to see if he might have gone there.

Sixty long minutes with no idea where our precious elder son was.

Had someone taken him? Was he being sold as a sex slave? Did he drown? Was he lost and panicked, looking for us?

Five minutes later, I saw him with Sallyann. He told us he had been in the water and had come out near our original setup area; he had waited there, lying on the sand. Sallyann found him as she returned from the hotel, where she had also alerted staff of his disappearance. I held his wet, swimsuit-clad body close and buried my face in his salty hair.

"I was right here, Mom. You were lost, not me," he chided.

He was right. At eleven, he knew I was lost without him.

It seems like yesterday as I remember Sawyer's eleven-year-old self, but here he is in front of me, and that was history now. A memory, but gone, and so must this stuff be gone in just four more days, I remind myself as I pick up a backpack from the shelf nearest me.

"How about this green backpack? The zipper is broken," I ask him.

"Yeah, toss it. Wait. Did you check it for stuff?" His wrinkled brow is showing.

"Yep, empty, all pockets," I assure him.

He looks longingly at the pile of boxes full of his favorite things, mostly books, ready for storage.

I respond to his look. "Let's take those up now. I will show you where all your stuff will be in the garage attic, closest to the door. We know you will want access to the books."

He smiles, both at that knowledge and that we know him.

"How about a Snapple break first?" I smile back at him.

"Yes!" he enthusiastically agrees.

We'd bought a case of his favorite drink to ease the burden of packing and to reward him for all the donkey-like traipsing up and down stairs, taking his and our stuff to the garage attic.

Each of us now has a corner in the attic: one shared by Sallyann and me, one for Sawyer, one for Seth's stuff, which is already there since he had to finish yesterday to get back to his apartment in Burlington. Then, the corner my eyes avoid, the corner furthest from the door of the attic, as if we are afraid it will creep out when we aren't there. The baby stuff. The things that still smell of Sage, if held close to the nose and heart. Sallyann still has the last sleeper and blanket that wrapped him from the cold fall air. It has lost its scent, really, but still somehow has his energy in its threads. To put it away is just too difficult, too painful to bear. How can we admit he isn't going to wear it ever again? That he won't be within these walls again?

On our last day with him, two friends came and took away the crib and changing table. Sallyann had sobbed, and I'd heard through the moans of pain that she did not want to see the furniture there when we returned from the lawyer's office, so I'd made the call. My sobs internal, my mouth and brain functional but numb, I called someone I trusted who'd not think it unreasonable. Meg and Tim had asked how they could help when they heard our horrific news. They were quick to agree, and when we got back from handing our precious boy over to the suit-clad lawyer, those two huge pieces of his existence in our home were gone. But so much was still there.

Sawyer helped trek everything except that blanket and sleeper out to the garage. Two other friends put it all up in the attic the next day. It burns my eyes to see it all. So much stuff to help love a baby: swing, bassinet, bouncer, clothes, blankets, diapers, bottles, burp pads, tiny sleepers that still need the sleeves rolled up to fit his little arms so his hands are free. He would be a thumb-sucker, like Sawyer, we were sure, as we watched him attempt to get fist to mouth.

Sawyer swigs down the last of his glass of raspberry Snapple and asks, "Ready?"

"No." I smile, with effort. "But let's get at it." Boxes fill up the space left near the doorway for his stuff in our trips up and down.

"Thanks again for setting up my girlfriend," he says with a grunt, putting down a large book-filled box, referring to Analise, and her move. Most of our furniture is headed to her new apartment because she is about to start her job in Vermont next week.

"No problem. It was logical, and perfect timing. We have stuff we don't need; she needs stuff." I reach out to pat his back and am surprised by a hug from him. He is a hugger, for sure, but I can feel his pain in all this and I am so sorry, so, so sorry that it is wrenchingly painful for us all. He is grateful to have Analise's apartment filled with not just furniture, but the familiar. He is a homebody, as independent as he is. Back in the living room he takes a break on his laptop, and I take a hammer and put up the trim that will cover the place in the doorway where pencil marks recorded the annual growth of Sawyer and Seth over the past fourteen years, one boy on each side of the doorway from kitchen to living room.

Sawyer had asked me, as he held Sage, "Where will we chart his growth?"

"In the doorway to the back hall, on the other side of the kitchen," I said as if I had planned it for years. In fact, I had.

Sallyann comes out of the bedroom where she has completely emptied the walk-in closet and all our bureau drawers. She looks at the progress on the trim.

"You are amazing." She smiles at me. A smile that is forced, but I appreciate her effort at joy, impossible right now. How can a smile and sob be so close together? So close they can be felt as one expression.

"No, you are," I reply, and return the smile.

As I start to cover the new trim with ivory paint, I see Sawyer's astonished stare.

"It is a new piece of wood. See?" I gesture to the trim. We are preparing the space for a friend who will be renting it from us.

For the past ten years, we'd had a loyal tenant upstairs. Now we would have one occupying *our* space, too.

"Your growth chart is still under there. These new pieces can be removed if we want."

We both know we never will.

EPILOGUE

Love will endure—if I can let you go

A SPIRAL OF EGGS
Sallyann, 2018

Rebecca and I decided we would share a squadron of chickens with our neighbors this summer. Since we are living back in the Northeast, we picked them up from a busy farm in Connecticut. They were just teenagers at the start of our nesting arrangement. And any day now, we expect to see them earn their keep by producing some eggs for us.

I look back on the events surrounding Sage and think, *How do I want them portrayed?* This is not just our story. It is also the story of everyone involved. It's just our rendition. It's the way we see it. I cannot rewrite these memories, and I'm not sure if the photocopied layers of my life are removed from the actual truth. Has the truth changed over time? Can truth change, or is it only our perception of it that changes?

The reality is that the people we write about—his birth mama, his grandma, and others—those are the people he will grow up with, the people he will develop his own truths about. They are the people he has depended on and come to love, pointy edges and all, like the rest of us. They are the family he knows and will remember.

In his life, we are the forgotten ones.

Truth can be gnarly. And so can loss. It can ache persistently and grow more painful over time, like arthritis. It can carry us on its rapids, descend, and throw us across a chasm. It's incongruous and can permeate places within us we don't know are there, like using a muscle that rarely gets exercised. When it does, we wonder—where did this feeling come from?

I understand our grief is synonymous with the love we felt: the greater the love, the more enveloping the grief. It sounds reasonable, but that makes me wary because, when it comes to grief, what do we make of reason? It operates separately, as if it is its own season.

And how in the world do you quantify love or loss? Do we count it by its effects on our lives? By the number of days we cry? Or by how we learn to stop crying? Can we even compare it against physical pain? Our arrogance promises that we could never feel the same pain again.

Now when I think about Sage, I think about the days his birth mother lost. I think about the pain that must come when she celebrates his birthday, or when others ask when he was born, and she must remember how she'd said she didn't want him. She must remember how she turned her head and refused to see him after he exited her body, how she refused to touch him in those first wondrous days of his life. I don't share her burden. When his birthday arrives, I recall the majesty of each moment we held him, looked into his newborn face, so inquisitive about the world where he'd landed. I remember the gift of closeness, of naked realness Rebecca and I shared with him in that hospital bed, excited about all the promise his life held.

I'm sure that when she let go of him, she didn't have

any awareness of all the consequences of her actions, any more than we do as we put this story out there. You can't know how any creation will be received. You can't completely estimate where the love goes when you give it away. You can't ever prepare for the pain that comes with the loss.

The gift of those days with him—I could never put a price tag on it. To believe he was our son—that was priceless. To treat him as our family that he belonged in, also beyond value. If you have ever felt that you didn't belong, it is difficult to describe just how powerful the relief of finding belonging is. To us, he fit. He belonged with us.

But the reality to me every day is that he is growing up belonging to other people. Delilah's reality could have been mine, if she'd kept her part in the unwritten contract that said, "Here, he is yours to love and raise now," and "I know you will uphold this agreement by taking care of him to the best of your ability."

We don't ever really know. We just have to trust that the intention and the outcome will reunite. Any contract, any bargain between people, falls into a chasm when trust breaks. Whether we lose trust in ourselves or the other hardly matters because, ultimately, all the unwritten rules we decode, all the dreams, hopes, and baggage we bring, drop into the depths.

When she planned to release him, I don't think Delilah's intention was ever to break our hearts. But I also think that her outcome never matched her intention, because she was never clear within herself. It's difficult to be clear, even when we embark on something and *think* we know what we want. We change, we learn, we grow; parts of us die. Often, we don't understand why.

There isn't a lot of room for that to happen in the best-written contracts we make, and there certainly isn't in the ones we break.

I'm still looking forward to what comes next. We will give our chickens space to grow, and tools for their curiosity, communication, and wholeness. Tomorrow, there will be eggs. And the next day, more eggs. We will share them with whomever is close by. We will wonder what they will be turned into, of the many shapes they could become.

And, hopefully, we will continue to give each other the space to grow as well.

ACKNOWLEDGMENTS

When we struggle, we read. It's one of the ways that we have grown as individuals and as a couple. When we experienced this tremendous loss, we searched the shelves and could not find a story that resonated with our inner and outer turbulence. When we need to heal, we write. We poured out our pain onto paper and in that process created the story that we needed. Yet this story could only come to fruition with the support and realization of the many people who supported us along the path.

We are especially grateful to the entire Rootstock team for believing in our story and its need to be delivered to the world.

Thank you to Patricia Brown for helping us build a love that was strong enough to sustain us.

Exceptional thanks to Linda Peavy and Ursula Smith for always believing we had a story worth telling.

To our readers and editors along the way who gave valuable input and insight, including Pat Jaquith, Helen Roby, and Sheryl Rapée-Adams, thank you for your time, energy, and attention to the many details.

Many thanks to John and Terry Walsh for giving us a place to land so we could sort out the initial tsunami of grief.

To our grown children, who made the desire for us to raise another child together so powerful, and for your flexibility in the aftermath.

Special thanks to all the people who believed in our journey and supported us along the way, including our dear friends and family, too numerous to list. Your compassion, generosity, and love continue to give us strength.

ABOUT THE AUTHORS

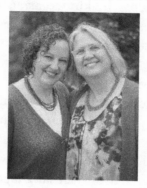

Rebecca Majoya received her bachelor's degree in education and theater arts and went on to receive her master's of education in curriculum design. She has been working as a homeschool consultant for the past twenty-eight years with homeschool families in Vermont. Rebecca has taught in public and private schools, grades K–12, and has created and taught classes in theater arts to homeschool kids, ages four to sixteen. She currently teaches at Community College of Vermont and works for Spectrum Youth & Family Services. She has over twenty-five years of social work experience, providing insight into what builds strong families and communities.

Sallyann Majoya's love of language began at an early age when she concocted elaborate fairy tales for her family, as well as stories of animal and child adventures. This led to her first degree in English, her work as a copywriter, grant writer, and editor. She served as an arts manager in a higher education setting, allowing her to marry her passion for arts and education, as she introduced students in kindergarten through college to world music, dance, and the liberal arts. Sallyann is also a certified therapeutic harpist who has brought a compassionate presence to a variety of hospice and palliative care environments. She holds an additional degree in wellness & alternative medicine and seeks to combine the principles of holistic health in helping others find a deeper, integrated sense of wellness through words and music. Currently, she is working to attain her graduate degree in speech-language pathology.

Also Available from Rootstock Publishing:

All Men Glad and Wise: A Mystery by Laura C. Stevenson

Alzheimer's Canyon: One Couple's Reflections on Living with Dementia by Jane Dwinell and Sky Yardley

The Atomic Bomb on My Back: A Life Story of Survival and Activism by Taniguchi Sumiteru

Blue Desert: A Novel by Celia Jeffries

Catalysts for Change: How Nonprofits and a Foundation are Helping Shape Vermont's Future by Doug Wilhelm

China in Another Time: A Personal Story by Claire Malcolm Lintilhac

Collecting Courage: Anti-Black Racism in the Charitable Sector Edited by Nneka Allen, Camila Vital Nunes Pereira, & Nicole Salmon

An Everyday Cult by Gerette Buglion

Fly with a Murder of Crows: A Memoir by Tuvia Feldman

Hawai'i Calls: A Novel by Marjorie Nelson Matthews

Horodno Burning: A Novel by Michael Freed-Thall

The Hospice Singer: A Novel by Larry Duberstein

I Could Hardly Keep from Laughing: An Illustrated Collection of Vermont Humor by Don Hooper & Bill Mares

The Inland Sea: A Mystery by Sam Clark

Intent to Commit: A Novel by Bernie Lambek

A Judge's Odyssey: From Vermont to Russia, Kazakhstan, and Georgia, Then on to War Crimes and Organ Trafficking in Kosovo by Dean B. Pineles

Junkyard at No Town: A Novel by J.C. Myers

The Language of Liberty: A Citizen's Vocabulary by Edwin C. Hagenstein

A Lawyer's Life to Live: A Memoir by Kimberly B. Cheney

Lifting Stones: Poems by Doug Stanfield

The Lost Grip: Poems by Eva Zimet

Lucy Dancer Story and Illustrations by Eva Zimet

No Excuses by Stephen L. Harris

Nobody Hitchhikes Anymore by Ed Griffin-Nolan

Pauli Murray's Revolutionary Life by Simki Kuznick

Preaching Happiness: Creating a Just and Joyful World by Ginny Sassaman

Red Scare in the Green Mountains: Vermont in the McCarthy Era 1946-1960 by Rick Winston

Safe as Lightning: Poems by Scudder H. Parker

Striding Rough Ice: Coaching College Hockey and Growing Up in the Game by Gary Wright

Street of Storytellers by Doug Wilhelm

Tales of Bialystok: A Jewish Journey from Czarist Russia to America by Charles Zachariah Goldberg

To the Man in the Red Suit: Poems by Christina Fulton

Uncivil Liberties: A Novel by Bernie Lambek

Venice Beach: A Novel by William Mark Habeeb

The Violin Family by Melissa Perley; Illustrated by Fiona Lee Maclean

Walking Home: Trail Stories by Celia Ryker

Wave of the Day: Collected Poems by Mary Elizabeth Winn

Whole Worlds Could Pass Away: Collected Stories by Rickey Gard Diamond

You Have a Hammer: Building Grant Proposals for Social Change by Barbara Floersch